AF524824

Practical Issues in Geriatrics

Series Editor
Stefania Maggi, Aging Branch, CNR-Neuroscience Institute, Padua, Italy

This practically oriented series presents state of the art knowledge on the principal diseases encountered in older persons and addresses all aspects of management, including current multidisciplinary diagnostic and therapeutic approaches. It is intended as an educational tool that will enhance the everyday clinical practice of both young geriatricians and residents and also assist other specialists who deal with aged patients. Each volume is designed to provide comprehensive information on the topic that it covers, and whenever appropriate the text is complemented by additional material of high educational and practical value, including informative video-clips, standardized diagnostic flow charts and descriptive clinical cases. Practical Issues in Geriatrics will be of value to the scientific and professional community worldwide, improving understanding of the many clinical and social issues in Geriatrics and assisting in the delivery of optimal clinical care.

Indexed in Scopus

Nicola Veronese • Anna Marseglia
Editors

Psychogeriatrics

A Clinical Guide

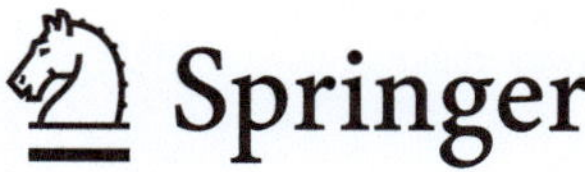

Editors
Nicola Veronese
Department of Geriatrics and Internal Medicine
University of Palermo
Palermo, Italy

Anna Marseglia
Department of Neurobiology
Care Sciences and Society
Division of Clinical Geriatrics
Karolinska Institute
Stockholm, Sweden

ISSN 2509-6060 ISSN 2509-6079 (electronic)
Practical Issues in Geriatrics
ISBN 978-3-031-58487-9 ISBN 978-3-031-58488-6 (eBook)
https://doi.org/10.1007/978-3-031-58488-6

This Springer imprint is published by the registered company Springer Nature Switzerland AG
The registered company address is: Gewerbestrasse 11, 6330 Cham, Switzerland

Preface

Welcome to the fascinating world of psychogeriatrics, a discipline devoted to understanding the complexity of mental health in aging. This book serves as a comprehensive guide to the multifaceted aspects of psychogeriatrics, providing insights into the psychological, biological, social, and ethical dimensions of mental health in older adults.

In recent years, the field of psychogeriatrics has gained increasing recognition and importance owing to the growing population of older adults globally. With advancements in healthcare and longer life expectancy, the number of older individuals confronting mental health challenges also is on the rise. Consequently, there is a pressing need for healthcare professionals, caregivers, researchers, and policymakers to deepen their understanding of psychogeriatric conditions, developing and implementing effective strategies for prevention, diagnosis, treatment, and care.

This book aims, to offer a comprehensive approach to psychogeriatrics, delving into a number of topics pertinent to mental health and aging. From dementia to prevalent psychiatric disorders in older adults, each chapter presents valuable insights and evidence-based recommendations. Furthermore, the book tackles key psychosocial and ethical aspects of caring for older individuals with mental health issues, such as the influence of social determinants of health, socio-cultural factors, and end-of-life care.

The contributors to this book are experts in the field of psychogeriatrics, comprising geriatricians, geriatric psychiatrists, neurologists, psychologists with background in aging and geriatrics, geriatric epidemiologists, and other healthcare professionals. Their diverse perspectives and wealth of experience enrich the content of this book, providing readers with a comprehensive and up-to-date resource for understanding and addressing the mental health needs of older adults.

Throughout the book, emphasis is placed on the importance of interdisciplinary collaboration and person-centered care in psychogeriatrics. Recognizing the unique needs and preferences of older individuals, as well as the complex interplay of psychological, social, and environmental factors, is essential for providing effective and compassionate care.

Beyond healthcare professionals, this book caters to caregivers, family members, undergraduate and graduate trainees, researchers, and anyone interested in learning more about psychogeriatrics. By raising awareness and knowledge of mental health issues in older adults, we can work together to promote healthy aging, enhance quality of life, and ensure dignity and respect for older individuals facing mental health challenges.

As editors, we are privileged to present this book as a valuable resource for advancing the field of psychogeriatrics and enhancing the care and support available to older adults with mental health needs. We hope that readers will find this book informative, thought-provoking, and ultimately empowering in their efforts to promote mental well-being and healthy aging in our aging population.

Sincerely

Palermo, Italy Nicola Veronese
Stockholm, Sweden Anna Marseglia

Contents

Anxiety and Depressive Disorders in Older Adults

1

Theodore D. Cosco, Megha Goel, Indira Riadi, Eliza R. Farquharson, Cari Randa, John Pickering, Jessica Miskiewicz, and John R. Best

1.1 Introduction

In this chapter, we seek to understand the complexities of depression and anxiety among older adults, a segment of the population frequently marginalized in mental health discourse. By recognizing that these mental health challenges are not uniform across life stages, this chapter specifically focuses on how they manifest, impact, and are addressed in older adulthood. We begin by dissecting the symptomatic profiles of depression and anxiety in this demographic, acknowledging the possibility that these conditions might represent either a continuation of lifelong mental health struggles or emerge as new challenges in later life. This distinction is crucial for developing appropriate therapeutic interventions and support systems.

The chapter further delves into the lived experiences of older adults living with depression and anxiety, highlighting how these conditions are intricately intertwined with the aging process. We explore the unique repercussions these mental health issues have on the quality of life, daily functioning, and overall well-being of older individuals. Special attention is given to the role of comorbidities, often prevalent in this age-group, which can complicate diagnosis and treatment. The interplay of physical health issues, such as cognitive decline and chronic illnesses, with

T. D. Cosco (✉)
School of Public Policy, Simon Fraser University, Vancouver, BC, Canada

Department of Gerontology, Simon Fraser University, Vancouver, BC, Canada

Oxford Institute of Population Ageing, University of Oxford, Oxford, UK
e-mail: theodore_cosco@sfu.ca

M. Goel · I. Riadi · C. Randa · J. Pickering · J. Miskiewicz · J. R. Best
Department of Gerontology, Simon Fraser University, Vancouver, BC, Canada

E. R. Farquharson
Division of Psychology and Language Sciences, University College London, London, UK

N. Veronese, A. Marseglia (eds.), *Psychogeriatrics*, Practical Issues in Geriatrics,
https://doi.org/10.1007/978-3-031-58488-6_1

mental health conditions, presents a layered challenge for healthcare providers and caregivers.

Moreover, we examine the psychological aspects, considering how life transitions, grief, and changes in social roles can contribute to or exacerbate mental health issues in older adults. The chapter also addresses the critical role of social factors, including isolation, socioeconomic status, and the evolving dynamics of family support in the mental health of the elderly. These factors are not only pivotal in understanding the prevalence and expression of depression and anxiety but also in shaping the approaches to treatment and care.

In discussing interventions, the chapter provides a balanced view of both pharmacological and non-pharmacological strategies. It emphasizes the importance of tailored treatment plans that consider the unique physiological responses of older adults to medication, alongside the potential benefits of psychotherapy, digital interventions, and community support systems. The goal is to present a holistic view of managing depression and anxiety in older adults, one that goes beyond mere symptom management to enhance overall life satisfaction and well-being.

By the end of this chapter, readers will gain a comprehensive understanding of the multifaceted nature of depression and anxiety in older adults. The insights offered aim to foster greater empathy, inform more effective treatment approaches, and ultimately improve the quality of life for older individuals grappling with these challenging mental health conditions.

1.2 Depression and Anxiety in the Context of Older Adults

Depression and anxiety are the most common mental health issues older adults may face in their lifetime. These two mental health problems may be lifelong, or with onset in older adulthood, with consequent repercussions pertaining to lived experiences and quality of life [1, 2]. Due to the interconnected nature of comorbid depression and anxiety, it can be difficult to separate onset of one disorder from the other; however, almost all anxiety disorders appear to show comorbidity with depressive symptoms of varying severity [1, 3]. The goals of the following section are twofold: (1) to introduce the symptomatic profiles of depression and anxiety in the context of older adults and (2) to explore the complexities of the lived experiences of older adults with depression and anxiety and the resulting multiple jeopardies when biological, psychological, and social factors interact.

1.2.1 Depression and Aging

Depression is not a normal part of the aging process; however, older adults are at an increased risk of developing depression over time. Although depression symptoms present similarly in older adults as with younger cohorts, older adults have the added burden of comorbid medical conditions including cognitive impairment and often receive ineffective treatment or symptoms even remain undetected [4].

Depressive symptoms accompany and interact with a wide array of experiences and comorbidities more common for older adults, so the indicators are easy to overlook and remain untreated, perpetuating negative perceptions of health and perceived futility of accessing health care services [5]. The bidirectional nature of depression and comorbid health conditions can occlude developing a holistic treatment plan. Major Depressive Disorder (MDD) and Persistent Depressive Disorder (PDD) are the two most common depressive disorders affecting older adults [6]. For more than half of people living with depression, onset of depressive symptoms is reported in older adulthood [7]. Although older adults appear to have lower prevalence of depression than younger cohorts, this can be explained with the survivorship bias, wherein those who are more severely affected die earlier. Even below diagnosable thresholds for Major Depressive Disorder (MDD), 10% to 15% of older adults experience clinically significant depressive symptoms [4, 8]. In community-dwelling older adults aged 65 and over, MDD ranges in prevalence 1–5% internationally, with most countries trending toward the lower range [7, 9].

1.2.2 Anxiety and Aging

The body of research is less robust exploring the symptoms, expression, and external factors characterizing anxiety disorders in older adults. As an explanation to the vast underreporting of anxiety disorders in older adults, these older adults may have withdrawn socially or are unable to cope with the multiple jeopardies of illnesses affecting all facets of their health and participation, especially to seek out and complete research opportunities. Anxiety disorders pertaining to older adults include specific phobias, social anxiety disorder, generalized anxiety disorder (GAD), panic disorder, and agoraphobia [6]. Prevalence of anxiety disorders in older adults is estimated to range from 3.2% to 14.2% [3, 6, 10]. Older adults living with anxiety later in life must overcome the detrimental effects of increased loneliness and isolation, decreased physical activity and associated health outcomes, and low satisfaction with perceived quality of life [11, 12]. Cognitive symptoms of anxiety like worry can exacerbate medical conditions and tax already frail physical defences.

1.3 Multiple Jeopardies

Aging is a multifaceted and complex human experience influenced by biological, psychological, and social factors, further complicated by mental health issues across the lifespan. It is important to note that adults living with chronic mental health issues, also referred to as serious persistent mental illness (SPMI), will have faced social exclusion, housing insecurity, and limited income potentially contributing to a lower subjective appraisal of the value of their life. Multimorbidities and similarities in expression of symptom present a difficult task for geriatric healthcare providers in making a differential diagnosis for appropriate treatment.

1.3.1 Biological Factors

Biological aging refers to natural, irreversible, and progressive age-related changes in metabolic chemical processes within the human body, diminishing regeneration at the cellular level and resulting in structural and functional changes [13]. Biological factors affect the location of interactions between older adults and kin or service providers as physical condition might dictate an older adult's location in the community, hospital, or long-term care [13]. Depression increases the risk of death in older adults living in long-term care 2–3 times more than those living in the community and exacerbates physical and cognitive decline [14]. Fiske et al. [7] suggest that insomnia is a ubiquitous risk factor for depression in older adults disrupting participation in daily activities and possibly contributing to negative thoughts about oneself. [3, 7]. Fostering understanding of psychiatric comorbidity of depression and anxiety is one option to engage interdisciplinary approaches to care for older adults [3]. The role of family history is less well understood for late onset depression and anxiety [3].

1.3.2 Psychological Factors

Psychological factors of aging include attitudes, awareness of, and adaptability to the aging process embedded within cultural norms [13]. Personality and individual coping styles contribute to negative thought patterns and pathways to accessing social support [3]. Older adults are more likely to experience transitions and losses, including grief and bereavement, in combination with other risk factors such as neuroticism as an enduring personality trait or a high medical burden with comorbid illnesses or caregiver stress as well as gender differences and hospitalization. Older adults are more likely to successfully take their own lives in association with depression than younger adults, due in part to increased baseline frailty higher than in younger adults and more closely associated with depression [6, 7]. In a systematic review, Beghi et al. [15] outline that older adults, especially white males over the age of 65, are at the highest risk for suicide due to the culmination of risk factors ranging from mental health issues, stress, bereavement, poor health, and isolation. Suicidal ideation can be challenging to identify for older adults, and better treatment of clinical depression for this population is an area in need of further research [16].

1.3.3 Social Factors

Marital status, income level, symptom expression, interpretation of illness, and response to disorder are connected to gender, with women developing depression, anxiety, or both later in life outnumbering men 2:1 [3, 7]. In addition, depression and anxiety may be experienced or expressed differently by varying ethnic groups but is need of further study for comparative representation. Globalization has dramatically changed family structure and expectations of intergenerational family care [17, 18]. Community support is a keystone for community-dwelling older adults because much of this population experiences a shrinking world with mobility, participation, and cognitive changes [17, 19]. In both developed and developing countries, older adults living in impoverished, isolated communities with limited social support, especially when children have moved away, experience the worst mental health outcomes [19–21]. Inequalities in housing, social support, income, and access to healthcare contribute to social determinants of health affecting quality of life and positive coping mechanisms influencing life satisfaction for older adults living with depression and anxiety [22].

1.4 Interventions for Depression and Anxiety

1.4.1 Pharmacological Interventions

1.4.1.1 Depression

For the initial treatment of depression, healthcare professionals may suggest a combination of antidepressant medication and psychotherapy. Well-designed studies have shown that combination treatment is more effective than either treatment on its own. Nevertheless, either treatment can also be given alone, as studies have also shown that each is effective and comparable to the other.

When selecting an antidepressant, it is important to consider the elderly patient's previous response to treatment, the type of depression, the patient's other medical problems, the patient's other medications, and the potential risk of overdose. Antidepressants are effective in treating depression in the face of medical illnesses, although caution is required so that antidepressant therapy does not worsen the medical condition or cause adverse events. For example, dementia, cardiovascular problems, diabetes, and Parkinson disease, which are common in the elderly, can worsen with highly anticholinergic drugs. Such drugs can cause postural hypotension and cardiac conduction abnormalities. It is also important to minimize drug–drug interactions, especially given the number of medications elderly patients are often taking. Tricyclic antidepressants are lethal in overdose and are avoided for this reason.

All the medications within a particular class are chemically related and function in a similar way. The more commonly used medications are from the following classes:

- Selective serotonin reuptake inhibitors (SSRIs) (Box 1.1)
- Serotonin-norepinephrine reuptake inhibitors (SNRIs)
- Atypical antidepressants
- Serotonin modulators

Box 1.1 SSRIs
Among the different antidepressants, SSRIs offer as much benefit as other medications with the least amount of risk in terms of safety and side effects. They are the most widely prescribed class of antidepressants. SSRIs—such as Lexapro, Celexa, Zoloft, Paxil and Prozac—are believed to alleviate symptoms of depression, excessive worry, and compulsivity by acting upon the brain's chemistry—specifically by blocking the breakdown and reabsorption of the neurotransmitter serotonin in the spaces between neurons. This selective reuptake inhibition causes serotonin levels to rise, promoting neuronal firing in circuits of the brain associated with mood and anxiety. SSRIs are all relatively safe in the elderly. They have lower anticholinergic effects than older antidepressants and are thus well tolerated by patients with cardiovascular disease. The alternatives to SSRIs include other second-generation antidepressants, namely serotonin-norepinephrine reuptake inhibitors, atypical antidepressants, and serotonin modulators.

Since all the second-generation antidepressants are roughly equivalent in terms of efficacy, health care providers select them based on other factors, such as:

- Each medication's safety and side effect profile
- The person's specific depressive symptoms
- Comorbid psychiatric and general medical illnesses
- The other medications the person is taking and whether they could interact with the chosen antidepressant
- Each medication's ease of use (for example, based on the number of pills the person must take each day)
- What the person prefers
- The cost of a medication and whether it is covered by insurance
- The person's previous responses to antidepressants (during past bouts of depression)

For example, for people who have trouble sleeping, health care providers often favor antidepressants known to promote sleep, such as mirtazapine. Similarly, for people who want to avoid the sexual side effects caused by many antidepressants, health care providers might favor bupropion, which is less likely to cause these side effects.

1.4.1.2 Anxiety

When treating anxiety disorders, antidepressants, particularly the SSRIs and some SNRIs (serotonin-norepinephrine reuptake inhibitors), have been shown to be effective.

Other anti-anxiety drugs include the benzodiazepines, such as as alprazolam (Xanax), diazepam (Valium), buspirone (Buspar), and lorazepam (Ativan). These drugs do carry a risk of addiction or tolerance (meaning that higher and higher doses become necessary to achieve the same effect), so they are not as desirable for long-term use. Other possible side effects include drowsiness, poor concentration, and irritability. Some anticonvulsant drugs (such as gabapentin [Neurontin] or pregabalin [Lyrica]), some blood pressure medications (such as propranolol), and some atypical antipsychotics (such as aripiprazole or quetiapine or Seroquel) are also occasionally used "off label" to treat anxiety symptoms or disorders.

1.4.1.3 Notable Points on Pharmacological Interventions

Dose—In general, health care providers tend to start their patients on low doses and slowly increase them as necessary. Once an antidepressant is selected for an older patient, the starting dose should be half that prescribed for a younger adult in order to minimize side effects. Increased side effects from antidepressant use in the elderly are thought to be due to changes in hepatic metabolism with aging, concurrent medical conditions, and drug–drug interactions. The best effects are often seen when doses are raised but still well tolerated.

How long before antidepressants take effect?—Antidepressants often take time to work, but many people start to feel better within 1–2 weeks. In fact, the people who see some benefit early on after starting an antidepressant appear to be the ones most likely to completely recover. That being said, it can take 6–12 weeks to see the full effect of an antidepressant, so health care providers may wait that long to make a final decision if a medication will be effective enough. If there is no significant improvement after 2–4 weeks on an average therapeutic dose, further increases should be made until there is either a clinical improvement, intolerable side effects, or the maximum suggested dose is reached. Thus, it is important to schedule regular follow-up visits to monitor treatment response while assessing for side effects and titrating accordingly.

1.4.2 Non-pharmacological interventions

1.4.2.1 Psychotherapy

All forms of psychotherapy include support from a professional who is focused on helping you to make positive psychological changes. There are many specific types of psychotherapy that are used to treat depression. Each works in a slightly different way, but all have been proven to help improve the symptoms of depression; many psychotherapists use a combination of techniques when working with clients (see Box 1.2).

Many forms of psychotherapy have been shown to be effective in the treatment of late-life depression, with similar efficacy rates achieved as found for younger and mid-life adults. The strongest evidence base exists for Problem Solving Therapy (PST) and Cognitive Behavior Therapy (CBT), with some evidence for Interpersonal Psychotherapy (IPT). A recent meta-analysis of psychotherapy for older adults found that, while the magnitude of effect depended on the type of control condition used, psychotherapy was overall effective in reducing depression. Increasing the availability of psychotherapy for older adults is especially crucial given consistent evidence that older adults prefer psychotherapy over medication to treat their depression. Despite these preferences, however, older adults rarely receive psychotherapy for depression due to a combination of access, availability, clinician workforce limitations, and individual-level factors like stigma.

Psychotherapy, as a non-pharmacological approach, plays a crucial role in treating depression and anxiety, offering professional support to facilitate positive psychological changes [23]. This form of treatment has shown to be equally effective in both older adults and younger populations, underscoring its versatility and broad applicability across different age-groups [24].

In the context of evidence-based therapeutic approaches for older populations, Cognitive Behavioral Therapies (CBTs), Problem Solving Therapy (PST), and Interpersonal Psychotherapy (IPT) stand out for their effectiveness. CBTs are particularly renowned for their well-documented success in treating a broad spectrum of mental and behavioral disorders. Additionally, PST offers a structured approach to problem-solving as a coping mechanism, while IPT focuses on improving interpersonal relationships. Despite the established efficacy of evidence-based therapy for treating depression and anxiety among older adults, research indicates that a relatively small proportion of this demographic actually pursue or have access to such therapy [25, 26].

Box 1.2 Forms of Psychotherapy

Cognitive and Behavioral Therapies (CBTs): CBT focuses on the interconnectedness of thoughts, feelings, and behaviors. The assumption is that negative thoughts and beliefs lead to emotional distress and maladaptive behavior. CBT posits that challenging detrimental thoughts and beliefs leads to changes in affect and behavior.

Behavioral Therapy (BT): A component of CBT primarily focuses on behavioral modification without the direct emphasis on cognition. This approach can be particularly suitable for older adults who have diminished cognitive abilities. BT focuses on enhancing positive behaviors, reducing avoidance patterns, and minimizing engagement in negative activities. It involves behavioral monitoring, where clients identify actions that lead to negative feelings and replace them with more enjoyable activities. Adjusting for any sensory or physical limitations to ensure full participation is essential in delivering effective BT, particularly for older adults.

Problem-Solving Therapy (PST): A structured approach that uses problem-solving as an active coping strategy. It consists of four stages: identifying the problem exacerbating depression, generating a list of potential solutions, evaluating these solutions and their consequences, and finally, implementing and assessing the effectiveness of the chosen solution. This approach is particularly beneficial for managing depressive symptoms, encouraging clients to actively tackle issues impacting their mental health.

Interpersonal Psychotherapy (IPT): The focus is on the client's relationships and social interactions. This therapy helps patients understand and improve their interactions with others, enhancing their social roles and relationships.

- CBT—In CBT, the patient works with a therapist to identify and reshape the thought and behavior patterns that contribute to their depression or anxiety.
- IPT—In interpersonal psychotherapy, the patient will focus on their relationships, the interactions with people in their lives, and the different social roles they play. In this form of psychotherapy, the patient can learn new ways to interact with others and improve existing and future relationships.
- PST—In problem-solving therapy, the patient takes a practical approach to the problem and decides on ways to solve them. For example, for a patient struggling with depression/anxiety due to financial struggles, they may work with a therapist to develop action steps to getting a job or budgeting.

1.4.2.2 Clinician Guided Self-help

For many older adults facing anxiety and mood disorders, a critical yet often overlooked step is recognizing their need for mental health care, which is vital for accessing necessary treatments and support. Enhanced efforts to educate both older adults and health professionals about the benefits and effectiveness of psychological therapies are essential to lower the barriers to seeking mental health care in this demographic [27].

For some older adults, engaging with a health professional might not be the most comfortable method to tackle their mental health issues. Instead of attending formal therapy sessions, they may opt to work on their own with limited guidance from a health care provider. Clinician guided self-help involves the use of workbooks (hardcopy, compact disc, or internet-based), audiotapes, or videotapes to monitor symptoms, changes in mood, and performing actions that can alleviate their depression/anxiety. People who choose this approach check in periodically with their health care provider but the interactions are much more brief and infrequent compared with formal therapy. Guided self-help can be a good choice for people who have mild depression and have no severe thoughts of self-harm or suicide.

1.4.2.3 Digital Mental Health Interventions

Digital mental health interventions are promising in their ability to provide researchers, mental health professionals, clinicians, and patients with personalized tools for assessing their behavior and seeking consultation, treatment, and peer support. A recent systematic review that examined existing randomized controlled trial studies on digital mental health interventions for older adults determined four factors that contributed to the success of digital mental health interventions: (1) ease of use; (2)

opportunities for social interactions; (3) having human support; and (4) having the digital mental health interventions tailored to the participants' needs.

Online therapy is the communication and relationship between clients and their mental health provider that is facilitated through online technology such as emails, videoconferencing, text messaging, and chat rooms [28]. For older populations, online therapy can offer significant logistical advantages, particularly in reducing the need for travel and increasing accessibility for those who might be far from treatment centers, face physical challenges in attending sessions, or have behavioral conditions that make traditional, in-person therapy less feasible [29]. Moreover, online therapy is recognized for its cost-effectiveness and ability to alleviate issues like long waiting lists [30].

Adding to the spectrum of digital mental health solutions, mental health apps are becoming increasingly crucial, especially for rural populations. These apps enhance the accessibility of care, allowing individuals to receive support anytime and anywhere, which is particularly beneficial in areas with limited mental health services [31]. The anonymity provided by these apps helps reduce the stigma often associated with seeking mental health care, making them a discreet option for those hesitant to seek traditional in-person therapy [31]. Furthermore, the affordability of these apps makes mental health care more accessible, addressing the economic barriers.

Many of these mobile applications are relatively easy to use and can be accessible by even older adults who are not technologically savvy. Older adults may have a preference to talk to a professional via phone call instead of through chat and an app that allows the user to choose the mode of communication can benefit a wider range of population. Examples of these smartphone applications are BetterHelp and Talkspace. The therapists on these therapy apps often have specific training in areas such as cognitive behavioral therapy, existential-humanistic approaches, dialectical behavioral therapy, psychodynamic, and mindfulness. The users of these apps can call, send text, video, and audio messages to their respected therapist at any time (https://www.betterhelp.com/; https://try.talkspace.com/).

Online CBT (iCBT): The effectiveness of Internet-delivered Cognitive Behavioral Therapy (iCBT) in alleviating symptoms of anxiety and depression among older adults has been well demonstrated in various studies [32]. In a study focusing on adults over 60 with symptoms of depression, iCBT interventions demonstrated significant improvements in reducing symptoms of both depression and anxiety [33]. These positive outcomes were not only observed post-treatment but also maintained at follow-up assessments conducted at 3 and 12 months, indicating the sustained effectiveness of the iCBT approach in this age-group [33].

Apps like Sanvello and MindShift provide web-delivered CBT for users with mild to moderate anxiety and depression. In a randomized study of 500 adults with mild to moderate anxiety and depression, online CBT apps like Sanvello were shown to decrease symptoms. In apps like Sanvello and Mindshift, there are also online communities that allow users to connect with others anonymously where people can share advice, ask questions, or talk to others who understand.

Online cognitive training has been shown to alleviate depressive and anxiety symptoms. An existing study used an online speed of processing training program on a group of older adults with early Alzheimer's disease. Their findings indicated that, through using the Geriatric Depression Scale, the training resulted in significant improvements in those who received the cognitive training compared with those in the waiting list group. Another recent online cognitive training study looked at a different cognitive training digital mental health intervention, recognized as a neuroplasticity-based computerized cognitive remediation, designed to target the cognitive control functions of older adults with late-life depression. The results showed that neuroplasticity-based computerized cognitive remediation induced remission in significant portions of the group

A study examined the effects of online Cognitive Training (CT) for older adults which reveals that such interventions can substantially improve cognitive abilities and the capacity to perform daily activities [34]. Notably, reasoning capabilities showed marked improvements, demonstrating the effectiveness of these online interventions. These advancements were on par with those achieved through traditional in-person training methods. This underscores the promise of online CT as a viable public health strategy, not only enhancing cognitive function in the elderly but also potentially reducing dementia risks.

1.4.2.4 Social Work and Mental Health Interventions

Social work approaches to treating mental health issues in older adults emphasize the influence of biological, psychological, and social factors. Social workers are unique among healthcare providers in that they are trained to work with the complexities of each individual's situation within the context of their environment [35]. Utilizing their understanding of systems theory and human behavior, social workers assist older adults in adapting to the changes that accompany the aging process, including managing loss and grief, addressing stress or worry, and rebuilding social networks [36]. The literature in aging research extensively documents the positive influence of social support in alleviating depression and nurturing a sense of purpose among older adults [37, 38]. Furthermore, sense of purpose, a central component of psychological well-being, has been linked to reduced risk for social anxiety, fewer depressive symptoms, and acts as a protective factor against depression-related cognitive decline in older adults [39–41].

For some diverse older adults, disruptions in family support and social harmony are identified as contributors to mental illness such as depression [42]. Geriatric social workers recognize the importance of involving family members in psychosocial and cognitive assessments and interventions. They help older adults and their support systems navigate complex behavioral health systems, coordinate care, and monitor service efficacy to provide comprehensive support [35]. The empathetic and holistic approach of social workers positions them as essential healthcare providers for older adults facing depression and anxiety, offering emotional support, disseminating information, facilitating connections, and empowering individuals. Moreover, incorporating the needs and concerns of the older person in mental health care decision-making is central to client-centered social work practice, fostering strong therapeutic relationships that are key predictors for help-seeking, treatment engagement, and adherence [43].

Geriatric social work encompasses various roles, ranging from acute healthcare to supportive social care [44]. Social workers contribute to multidisciplinary healthcare teams, engage in community-based case management, and provide clinical services such as crisis intervention and counseling [35]. Additionally, social workers conduct functional assessments of older people's everyday competence, positioning them well to observe nuanced changes in daily mental and cognitive functioning [35]. Recognizing symptoms based on changes in daily habits enables social workers to intervene early [45]. Addressing physical limitations and long-term care needs arising from depression and anxiety symptoms is another crucial aspect of geriatric social work, involving connecting older adults to home health services for their medical, functional, and social well-being. Supportive care becomes especially beneficial for older adults with anxiety disorders and cognitive impairments that may lead to isolation.

Social workers play a pivotal role in addressing challenges to the quality of life of older adults with mental health issues through direct practice as well as meso/macro level work. They advocate for social justice, human rights, and equal access to mental health services throughout old age [46].

1.5 Summary

This chapter provides an exploration of depression and anxiety among older adults, shedding light on the multifaceted nature of these mental health challenges. It delves into the symptomatic profiles, the impact of comorbidities, and the unique lived experiences of older individuals grappling with these conditions. The discussion underscores the importance of recognizing the distinct ways in which depression and anxiety manifest in older adulthood, influenced by a complex interplay of biological, psychological, and social factors. The chapter emphasizes the critical need for tailored interventions, advocating for a holistic approach that encompasses both pharmacological and non-pharmacological strategies to address the specific needs of this demographic. By highlighting the role of psychotherapy, digital interventions, and the invaluable support of social work, the chapter aims to foster a deeper understanding of the challenges faced by older adults with depression and anxiety. Ultimately, it calls for greater empathy, informed treatment approaches, and enhanced support systems to improve the quality of life for older individuals facing these profound mental health issues, advocating for a society that better accommodates the mental health needs of its aging population.

References

1. Cameron OG. Understanding comorbid depression and anxiety. Psychiatric Times. 2007;24(14):51. https://www.psychiatrictimes.com/view/understanding-comorbid-depression-and-anxiety. Accessed 24 Aug 2022.
2. Cameron OG, Abelson JL, Young EA. Anxious and depressive disorders and their comorbidity: effect on central nervous system noradrenergic function. Biol Psychiatry. 2004;56(11):875–83. https://doi.org/10.1016/j.biopsych.2004.08.007.

3. Beattie E, Pachana NA, Franklin SJ. Double jeopardy: comorbid anxiety and depression in late life. Res Gerontol Nurs. 2010;3(3):209–20. https://doi.org/10.3928/19404921-20100528-99.
4. Kok RM, Reynolds CF. Management of depression in older adults: a review. JAMA. 2017;317(20):2114–22. https://doi.org/10.1001/jama.2017.5706.
5. World Health Organization. Mental health of older adults; 2017, December 17. https://www.who.int/news-room/fact-sheets/detail/mental-health-of-older-adults. Accessed 22 Aug 2022.
6. Segal DL, Qualls SH, Smyer MA. Aging and mental health. Hoboken: Wiley; 2018. p. 207–312.
7. Fiske A, Wetherell JL, Gatz M. Depression in older adults. Annu Rev Clin Psychol. 2009;5:363. https://doi.org/10.1146/annurev.clinpsy.032408.153621.
8. Blazer DG. Depression in late life: review and commentary. J Gerontol Ser A Biol Med Sci. 2003;58(3):M249–65. https://doi.org/10.1093/gerona/58.3.m249.
9. Hasin DS, Goodwin RD, Stinson FS, Grant BF. Epidemiology of major depressive disorder: results from the National Epidemiologic Survey on Alcoholism and Related Conditions. Arch Gen Psychiatry. 2005;62(10):1097–106. https://doi.org/10.1001/archpsyc.62.10.1097.
10. Wolitzky-Taylor KB, Castriotta N, Lenze EJ, Stanley MA, Craske MG. Anxiety disorders in older adults: a comprehensive review. Depress Anxiety. 2010;27(2):190–211. https://doi.org/10.1002/da.20653.
11. Fuentes K, Cox B. Assessment of anxiety in older adults: a community-based survey and comparison with younger adults. Behav Res Ther. 2000;38(3):297–309. https://doi.org/10.1016/s0005-7967(99)00067-4.
12. Wetherell JL, Thorp SR, Patterson TL, Golshan S, Jeste DV, Gatz M. Quality of life in geriatric generalized anxiety disorder: a preliminary investigation. J Psychiatr Res. 2004;38(3):305–12. https://doi.org/10.1016/j.jpsychires.2003.09.003.
13. Dziechciaz M, Filip R. Biological psychological and social determinants of old age: Bio-psycho-social aspects of human aging. Ann Agric Environ Med. 2014;21(4) https://doi.org/10.5604/12321966.1129943.
14. Canadian Psychological Association. "Psychology Works" Fact Sheet: Depression among seniors. 2014. http://www.cpa.ca/docs/File/Publications/FactSheets/PsychologyWorksFactSheet_DepressionAmongSeniors.pdf. Accessed 22 Aug 2022
15. Beghi M, Butera E, Cerri CG, Cornaggia CM, Febbo F, Mollica A, Berardino G, Piscitelli D, Resta E, Logroscino G, Daniele A, Altamura M, Bellomo A, Panza F, Lozupone M. Suicidal behaviour in older age: a systematic review of risk factors associated to suicide attempts and completed suicides. Neurosci Biobehav Rev. 2021;127:193–211. https://doi.org/10.1016/j.neubiorev.2021.04.011.
16. Draper BM. Suicidal behaviour and suicide prevention in later life. Maturitas. 2014;79(2):179–83. https://doi.org/10.1016/j.maturitas.2014.04.003.
17. Benjamin D, Brandt L, Fan JZ. Ceaseless toil? Health and labor supply of the elderly in rural China. Health and Labor Supply of the Elderly in Rural China (June 2003). 2003. https://doi.org/10.2139/ssrn.417820
18. Song Q. Facing "double jeopardy"? Depressive symptoms in left-behind elderly in rural China. J Aging Health. 2017;29(7):1182–213. https://doi.org/10.1177/0898264316659964.
19. Kubzansky LD, Subramanian SV, Kawachi I, Fay ME, Soobader MJ, Berkman LF. Neighborhood contextual influences on depressive symptoms in the elderly. Am J Epidemiol. 2005;162:253–60. https://doi.org/10.1093/aje/kwi185.
20. Galea S, Ahern J, Nandi A, Tracy M, Beard J, Vlahov D. Urban neighborhood poverty and the incidence of depression in a population-based cohort study. Ann Epidemiol. 2007;17:171–9. https://doi.org/10.1016/j.annepidem.2006.07.008.
21. Ross CE. Neighborhood disadvantage and adult depression. J Health Soc Behav. 2000;41:177–87. https://doi.org/10.2307/2676304.
22. Silveira ER, Ebrahim S. Social determinants of psychiatric morbidity and well-being in immigrant elders and whites in east London. Int J Geriatr Psychiatry. 1998;13(11):801–12. https://doi.org/10.1002/(sici)1099-1166(1998110)13:11<801::aid-gps876>3.0.co;2-z.

23. Raue PJ, McGovern AR, Kiosses DN, Sirey JA. Advances in Psychotherapy for Depressed Older Adults. Curr Psychiatry Rep. 2017;19(9):57. https://doi.org/10.1007/s11920-017-0812-8. PMID: 28726061; PMCID: PMC6149527.
24. Cuijpers P, van Straten A, Warmerdam L, Andersson G. Psychotherapy versus the combination of psychotherapyand pharmacotherapy in the treatment of depression: a meta-analysis. Depress Anxiety. 2009;26(3):279–88. https://doi.org/10.1002/da.20519.
25. Peng X-D, Huang C-Q, Chen L-J, Lu Z-C. Cognitive behavioural therapy and reminiscence techniques for thetreatment of depression in the elderly: a systematic review. J Int Med Res. 2009;37: 975–82.
26. Mackenzie CS, Reynolds K, Cairney J, Streiner DL, Sareen J. Disorder-specific mental health service use for moodand anxiety disorders: associations with age, sex, and psychiatric comorbidity. Depress Anxiety. 2012;29:234–42.
27. Wuthrich VM, Frei J. Barriers to treatment for older adults seeking psychological therapy. International Psychogeriatrics. 2015;27(7):1227–36. https://doi.org/10.1017/S1041610215000241.
28. Cipolletta S, Damiano M. Online counseling: An exploratory survey of Italian psychologists' attitudes towards new ways of interaction†. Psychotherapy Research. 28 2018;909–24.
29. Kruse C, Fohn J, Wilson N, et al. Utilization barriers and medical outcomes commensurate with the use of telehealth among older adults: Systematic review. JMIR Med Inform. 2020;8(8):e20359.
30. Guzman D, Ann-Yi S, Bruera E, Wu J, Williams JL, Najera J, Raznahan M, Carmack CL. Enhancing palliative care patient access to psychological counseling through outreach telehealth services. Psychooncology. 2020;29(1):132–8. https://doi.org/10.1002/pon.5270.
31. Wright JH, Chan SR, Mishkind MC. Practical considerations for emerging types of telebehavioral health care: computer-assisted cognitive behavior therapy and mobile applications. In Virtual Mental Health Care for Rural and Underserved Settings. Cham: Springer International Publishing. 2020. pp. 145–64.
32. Spek V, Cuijpers P, Nyklicek I, Riper H, Keyzer J, Pop V. Internet-based cognitive behaviour therapy for symptoms of depression and anxiety: a meta-analysis. Psychol Med. 2007;37:319–28.
33. Titov N, Dear BF, Ali S, Zou JB, Lorian CN, Johnston L, ... Fogliati VJ. Clinical and costeffectiveness of therapist-guided internet-delivered cognitive behavior therapy for older adults with symptoms of depression: a randomized controlled trial. Behavior therapy, 2015;46(2):193–205.
34. Corbett A, Owen A, Hampshire A, Grahn J, Stenton R, Dajani S, ... Ballard C. The effect of an online cognitive training package in healthy older adults: an online randomized controlled trial. JAMA. 2015;16(11):990–7.
35. Greene RR., Choi N. Gerontology: a field of practice. In: Comprehensive handbook of social work and social welfare, the profession of social work, vol 1; 2008. p. 283
36. Ray M, Milne A, Beech C, Phillips J, Richards S, Sullivan MP, Tanner D, Lloyd L. Gerontological social work: reflections on its role, purpose and value. Br J Soc Work. 2015;45(4):1296–312. https://doi.org/10.1093/bjsw/bct195.
37. Liu L, Gou Z, Zuo J. Social support mediates loneliness and depression in elderly people. J Health Psychol. 2016;21(5):750–8. https://doi.org/10.1177/1359105314536941.
38. Son H, Cho HJ, Cho S, Ryu J, Kim S. The moderating effect of social support between loneliness and depression: differences between the young-old and the old-old. Int J Environ Res Public Health. 2022;19(4):2322. https://doi.org/10.3390/ijerph19042322.
39. Lewis NA, Hill PL. Sense of purpose promotes resilience to cognitive deficits attributable to depressive symptoms. Front Psychol. 2021;12:698109. https://doi.org/10.3389/fpsyg.2021.698109.
40. Kashdan TB, McKnight PE. Commitment to a purpose in life: an antidote to the suffering by individuals with social anxiety disorder. Emotion (Washington, D.C.). 2013;13(6):1150–9. https://doi.org/10.1037/a0033278.
41. Windsor TD, Curtis RG, Luszcz MA. Sense of purpose as a psychological resource for aging well. Dev Psychol. 2015;51(7):975–86. https://doi.org/10.1037/dev0000023.

42. Jimenez DE, Bartels SJ, Cardenas V, Dhaliwal SS, Alegría M. Cultural beliefs and mental health treatment preferences of ethnically diverse older adult consumers in primary care. Am J Geriatr Psychiatry. 2012;20(6):533–42. https://doi.org/10.1097/JGP.0b013e318227f876.
43. Polacsek M, Boardman GH, McCann TV. Help-seeking experiences of older adults with a diagnosis of moderate depression. Int J Ment Health Nurs. 2019;28(1):278–87. https://doi.org/10.1111/inm.12531.
44. Gonyea JG, Hudson RB, Curley A. The geriatric social work labor force: challenges and opportunities in responding to an aging society. Public Policy Aging Rep. 2004;13(2):12–6. https://doi.org/10.1093/ppar/13.2.12.
45. McCrae N, Murray J, Banerjee S, Huxley P, Bhugra D, Tylee A, Macdonald A. 'They're all depressed, aren't they?' A qualitative study of social care workers and depression in older adults. Aging Ment Health. 2005;9(6):508–16. https://doi.org/10.1080/13607860500193765.
46. International Federation of Social Workers. World Mental Health Day: The crucial role of social workers in advancing mental well-being; 2023. https://www.ifsw.org/world-mental-health-day-the-crucial-role-of-social-work-in-advancing-mental-well-being/.

2 Bipolar Disorder in Older People

Laura Montejo and Andrea Murru

2.1 Definition and Epidemiology

Bipolar disorder (BD) is a mood disorder, characterized by acute episodes of depression and (hypo)mania, affecting approximately 2.4% of the global population [1]. Previous studies have shown that there is considerable functional impairment in adults with BD, even while their mood is stable [2–4]. Similarly, studies have found that quality of life is impaired when individuals are both in episode and euthymic [5, 6]. For these reasons, BD has been ranked as one of the top 20 causes of the global disease burden [7]. As BD represents a lifelong and recurrent condition, associated with functional decline and a reduction in quality of life [6, 8], people suffering from it nowadays live most of their life with this disorder.

Within the general population, recent epidemiological studies indicate that approximately 0.5–1% of older adults have a diagnosis of BD [9]. This percentage is slightly lower than that observed in younger individuals, among whom the esteemed prevalence is 2% [9]. These demographic changes mean that this population will increasingly constitute a higher percentage within BD and general geriatric population, increasing the importance of paying specific attention to them. To date, approximately 25% of all patients with BD are aged 60 years and over [10], and this was esteemed to possibly increase to 50% in 2030 [11]. On the other hand, until a few decades ago, the study of Older Adults with Bipolar Disorder (OABD) and their possible unique needs had been neglected, with many international guidelines considering this group of patients as a "special subpopulation" that require no or small specific recommendations for assessment and management [12]. In recent years, the task force for Older Adults with Bipolar Disorder was created by the *International Society of Bipolar Disorders (ISBD)* [12] in which OABD was

L. Montejo · A. Murru (✉)
Bipolar and Depressive Disorders Unit, IDIBAPS CIBERSAM, Hospital Clinic, Barcelona, Spain
e-mail: lmontejo@recerca.clinic.cat; amurru@clinic.cat

N. Veronese, A. Marseglia (eds.), *Psychogeriatrics*, Practical Issues in Geriatrics,
https://doi.org/10.1007/978-3-031-58488-6_2

defined as people with BD over the age of 50. Henceforth, special emphasis has been placed on the need to consider OABD as a population subgroup requiring specific approaches, as they present differential characteristics in terms of clinical profile, medical and psychiatric comorbidities, cognitive performance, and psychosocial functioning compared to younger BD adults. For these reasons, results from younger cohorts cannot be directly extrapolated to the older population, but rather clinical and research strategies specifically designed for OABD must be conducted.

2.2 Clinical Profile of OABD

Within the BD course, the clinical profile of the illness may change with time. In general, while some studies suggest that an overall decrease in symptom severity as age advances [13], other aspects directly and indirectly related with the illness do become more important, such as medical comorbidities and cognitive impairment [12, 14, 15].

According to the literature on disease course, in OABD, a more prevalent recurrence toward depression than mania was described [16, 17], but a possible increased risk to recurrences, although somewhat milder (i.e., not leading to admissions) was also outlined [18, 19]. Coherently, OABD analysis from a large international cohort detected a decrease in the severity of both manic and subsyndromal depressive symptoms with advancing age [15] indicating less severity of BD symptoms in older compared to younger adult patients. Regarding to mental health and overall health access and use, while the number of hospitalizations for illness recurrences is lower in the elderly [18], the duration of hospital admissions is increased [20], as well as, the use of tertiary resources, as increased medium-long stay admissions in social-health centers and nursing homes are frequently needed [21].

Similarly, a lower prevalence of prevalence of psychotic symptoms is also noted as age advances [16, 22]. Mixed symptoms become more predominant in the illness course of OABD, and are strongly associated with poor functioning [23]. Functional recovery after an episode relapse is slower and takes longer due to more frequent medical and cognitive complications [24]. However, the illness subtype of affective disorder diagnosis (BD-I vs BD-II) does not differ in terms of cognitive outcomes, functioning, and somatic burden in OABD, altough BD-II tends to present a later age of onset and more severe depressive recurrence [25].

Suicidal behaviors in OABD are far less studied. Within the suicide curve distribution, a convex trend is observed, with high suicide rates found in both young and older patients, and a decline in middle-aged BD adults [26, 27]. The importance of treatment adherence seems pivotal, as a lower risk of suicide in older patients positively relates with a good adherence to pharmacological treatment [28], even when the disorder began with early onset [13].

It is important to emphasize that the results of some OABD studies may be biased due to the “survival cohort effect”. This concept suggests that BD patients who reach older age may have more resilient traits to withstand the impact of the disease, and it even proposes that a more benign disease phenotype might underlie patients' survival. Even so, when compared to older individuals without BD, older patients with BD show biological markers of premature aging and accelerated brain aging, which represent conditions that may nonetheless lead to premature death and decreased life expectancy. Specifically, markers of premature aging include both biological factors, such as telomere length, DNA methylation, inflammation, and oxidative stress, and environmental factors such as childhood trauma, lifestyle habits, psychological stress, among others [29, 30]. The illness has an effect, even long term, on the brain structure, as BD patients show faster enlargement of ventricular volumes and slower thinning of the fusiform and parahippocampal cortex, especially associated with relapses toward mania [31].

As age advances, clinical manifestations of BD change toward a less intense, more predominantly depressive course of illness, with an increased risk of suicide, strongly reduced when OABD is appropriately treated. Medical comorbidities and cognitive impairment, with a subsequent overall reduction in functioning and autonomy, may complicate the duration of the otherwise less frequent acute episodes needing an hospitalization [15].

2.3 Somatic Comorbidities

Somatic comorbidities are more frequent in OABD patients compared to general age-stratified population and also compared to younger adults with BD [15, 17, 32]. On average, patients with OABD present 3–4 somatic comorbidities, including hypertension, metabolic syndrome, cardiovascular disease, diabetes mellitus, endocrine abnormalities, arthritis, and respiratory diseases, among others [12, 32–35]. Sex differences in number and type of somatic comorbidities have also been observed [36]. OABD women exhibit more respiratory, gastrointestinal, musculoskeletal, and endocrinological diseases than men. Moreover, men with OABD tend to have more cardiovascular, renal, and endocrinological comorbidities than men without OABD [36].

Longitudinally, OABD patients show a faster accumulation of chronic physical illnesses and less health perceptions compared with the general population, a finding that, at least in part, may stem from variations in psychosocial factors, lifestyle choices, and healthcare behaviors [37]. Taken together, these findings highlight the increased complexity of clinical management for OABD patients, who may frequently require multiple medications. In fact, promoting measures that encourage a healthy lifestyle such as physical exercise, a balanced diet, or stress coping strategies, could reduce the impact of these comorbid diseases [38]. Therefore, integrating these psychosocial and behavioral recommendations into the therapeutic plan of OABD patients should be a routine practice.

2.4 Age of Onset: Differences Between OABD Early and Late Onset

OABD presents heterogeneity according to age of onset, with both *early onset* and *late onset* being possible. Although there is no established consensus regarding the cut-off point for the age of onset within OABD, most authors set it at 50 years [12]. An *early onset bipolar disorder* (EOBD) is defined by the onset of the first episode—mania/hypomania, depression, or both—before the age of 50. Conversely, the new onset of mania/hypomanic episode after the age of 50 without any previous depressive episodes, it is defined as *late-onset bipolar disorder* (LOBD). Within OABD, the estimated prevalence of LOBD ranged from 5% to 17% [10, 39]. Patients who experienced a first manic/hypomanic episode after the age of 50 years but had previously presented at least one depressive episode in adulthood (<50 years) are defined within the conceptual framework of "*conversion to bipolar disorder*" *or late-onset mania*.

Some recent evidence indicates that these two groups present distinct characteristics, differing, for example, in etiology, neurobiological factors, clinical symptoms, cognitive performance, and medical comorbidities, among others [12, 14, 40]. Therefore, the age at onset might bear important clinical and prognostic implications. While factors associated with the development of EOBD would be more related to a family history of psychiatric history, especially with family history of mood disorders [41], LOBD would be associated with cerebrovascular diseases. In neuroimaging studies, LOBD presents white matter alterations such as increased hyperintense signals and an increased risk for stroke compared with EOBD and healthy controls [42, 43]. This suggests that cerebrovascular risk plays an important role in the clinical expression of LOBD. Although the number of studies is limited, it seems that patients with LOBD show a more progressive disease course, an increased risk of episode recurrence [12] and greater medical and neurological burden [44, 45]. Despite the shorter duration of the disease, a late onset is associated with greater severity of cognitive impairment compared to OEBD patients [46]. Contrary to these findings, some evidence has not found such marked differences based on age at onset. Recently, although limited by its retrospective design, a study using data from an international consortium found no significant differences in terms of clinical symptomatology (depression or mania) or psychosocial functioning, thus supporting the hypothesis that LOBD might represent a similar clinical phenotype as EOBD [47].

Taken together, these findings highlight the idea whether both groups constitute two sides of the same coin under the same diagnostic entity, differing in the form of presentation; or, on the contrary, they constitute two different clinical entities with different etiology but show such a similar "phenotype" that can be easily classified under the same diagnostic umbrella. Future longitudinal studies and analysis of neurobiological and biomarker factors may provide more accurate data to help clarify this question.

2.5 Neurocognition

Cognitive dysfunction is prevalent in adults BD, and studies focused on younger population (with a mean age of 40 years old) report impairments in memory, attention, executive functions, and processing speed [48–50]. Not surprisingly, these cognitive deficits have been found to persist into advanced ages. A recent meta-analysis focused in OABD has identified impairment in many cognitive domains such as verbal memory, working memory, processing speed, attention, and executive functions, showing large and moderate effect sizes [51]. Nevertheless, cognitive heterogeneity has been identified in OABD based on the severity of cognitive dysfunction. In fact, not all patients exhibit cognitive impairment with the same severity. Specifically, almost half of the patients (46%) show cognitive performance similar to healthy controls, another similar percentage (42%) exhibit mild cognitive impairment and, a smaller proportion of OABD patients (12%) show severe cognitive impairment in attention, memory, processing speed, executive functions, and working memory [52].

Although neurocognition on OABD represents a field with heterogeneous and inconclusive evidence, efforts have been made to identify the associations of age-related variables with cognitive function. Some disease-specific factors such as number of admissions, late onset, and higher number of manic episodes as well as the presence of vascular risk factors represent established factors associated with worse cognitive performance, especially with memory, attention, and executive functions [44].

Overall, OABD is a population vulnerable to cognitive decline, since they present the effect of a *double burden* determined by, on the one hand, the cumulative factors of the disease, and, on the other hand, the paraphysiological effects of a normal aging process. The neuroprogression hypothesis postulates that the cognitive decline in BD would be the result of some disease events, such as number and type of episodes (especially manic episodes), illness duration, and number of admissions [53–55]. Thus, each specific "stressful" event of the disease would favor subsequent cognitive decline as certain neurotoxic processes occur through mechanisms that include the accumulation of factors contributing to an overall increased allostatic load, such as oxidative stress and an altered imbalance of neurotrophins/pro-inflammatory mediators, all contributing to structural and functional brain changes and, ultimately, neurodegeneration [54, 56]. Yet, as previously outlined, disease progression in terms of cognitive and functional outcomes is not an inevitable and homogeneous outcome in the illness course or for all patients, as heterogeneous trajectories have been supported [57, 58].

The evolution of cognitive performance within illness progression in BD is not clear. Some longitudinal studies show a general trend toward no significant accelerated cognitive decline in BD compared with healthy controls [59, 60]. Likewise, a recent meta-analysis [61] that included longitudinal studies comparing cognitive performance between a recent-onset BD versus late-life BD—with an early onset group—patients did not found conclusive evidence of cognitive decline at 2 years follow-up, pointing to a possible discriminant effect operated by earlier, neurodevelopmental factors.

On the other hand, one study analyzing global neuropsychological performance with a dementia screening battery did detect that the group of OABD patients had more cognitive dysfunction and faster cognitive decline compared to HC [62]. Similarly, a sample of BD-I patients ranging from adult to OABD identified a significant age-associated cognitive decline in the processing speed domain, while the remaining cognitive domains remained stable throughout the life span [63]. Likewise, another cross-sectional study identified a significant age X group interaction concerning executive functions [64]. Finally, a cross-sectional study that included a large sample of BD between the ages of 18 and 80 years observed a significant decline in attentional-processing speed ability associated with BD and older age [65]. These latter findings would point to the presence of a specific selective cognitive decline in specific cognitive functions associated with age and BD, rather than a generalized deterioration of cognitive function.

Finally, there is also evidence that a subgroup of BD patients shows a worse evolution of cognitive performance [54, 58]. Importantly, an increased risk of dementia has been associated with history of mood disorders, especially BD patients exhibit higher risk compared to the general population and to major depressive disorder [66–68]. In addition, the number of affective episodes involving hospital admissions seems to be a predictor for the development of dementia in BD [69], and lithium treatment has been identified as a protective factor against diagnosis of dementia [67].

Given these evidence, the question arises whether dementia in BD occurs as a late stage of cognitive impairment, as an underlying process of disease course, or it stems as a comorbid condition with an increased risk in BD, or both aspects somehow coexist [70]. Interestingly, when Alzheimer's dementia (AD) biomarkers, such as beta-amyloid accumulation or TAU protein, have been investigated in BD, no evidence of increased concentrations in BD patients have been found. This allows concluding that cognitive impairment in BD does not have the AD pathophysiological features and alternate underlying mechanisms should be clarified [71]. Likewise, when OABD have been compared with patients with behavioral variant frontotemporal dementia (bv-FTD), the latter exhibited worse cognitive performance in executive functions and social cognition, but also greater signs of brain atrophy in frontal, temporal and parietal areas [72]. Of note, approximately a 50% of patients with bv-FTD had a prior psychiatric diagnosis, with a significant symptomatic overlap with BD [73].

To conclude, OABD patients represent a good opportunity to study the evolution of cognitive functions and decline as the disease progresses. Cognitive performance in BD presents heterogeneous trajectories, and this variability observed between patients may depend not only on disease-related associated clinical factors but may also be related to previous history and environmental factors such as cognitive reserve, healthy lifestyle habits, etc. This fuels the opportunity to design preventive intervention strategies against cognitive deterioration, focused on a systematic approach and treatment of those factors which appear potentially modifiable.

2.6 Psychopharmacological Treatment

When considering the pharmacological treatment of OABD, several general aspects must be taken into account, such as changes in age-related pharmacokinetic and pharmacodynamic characteristics (such as distribution volume, protein binding, metabolism, reduced enzyme activities). This frequently translates into using overall lower doses among elderly patients.

Special attention must be paid to CYP3A4, which represents the main metabolic pathway of frequently used antidepressants such as sertraline and citalopram, diminishes with age. Of note, however, there appears to be minimal age-related changes in CYP2D6 function which is relevant for metabolizing several other antidepressants, such as several tricyclics, fluoxetine, and the SNRIs duloxetine and venlafaxine [74]. Also, adverse drug reactions increase with age, even at lower drug concentrations, including dizziness, and sedation [74]. Last, and logically, in OABD, an elevated probability of drug interactions exists given the larger number of medications taken, and an increased number of medications may also cause difficulties with adherence, either due to lack of insight or cognitive impairment.

Lithium is considered an effective therapy for manic and depressive episodes and relapse prevention of bipolar disorders [14, 75]. In a single controlled trial in acute mania (vs. valproic acid), lithium was superior to valproic acid in YMRS score change from baseline (P <0.001 at endpoint (week 9), especially in severely manic patients (with scores at YMRS >30) [76]. In a post hoc analysis of the maintenance studies, lithium significantly delayed time to intervention for mania/hypomania/mixed episode in comparison to placebo, but not for time to intervention for depression [12]. So, a treatment trial with lithium can be recommended, and as the distribution volume is higher in old age, but the renal clearance is reduced, a lower dose of one-third to one-half should be used [40]. The risk of potential kidney dysfunction in lithium-treated BD patients represents a source of major concern in clinical practice and becomes an issue of uttermost importance in a population with high rates of physical comorbidities such as OABD. In different studies, an approximate 25% possibility of impaired kidney function is reported [77], but the actual occurrence of severe renal disfunction is definitely rare [78].

The efficacy of valproic acid has been only tested in the already cited controlled trial against lithium [76], with valproic acid showing inferior response compared to lithium. There are no controlled maintenance data for valproic acid in old age BD, and data from adult age trials are inconclusive [79].

The potential dementia-facilitating effect of valproate and lithium in a population of 4784 OABD (50+ years) has been studied. The risk for dementia was assessed between valproate-only, lithium-only, and combined valproate-lithium users, lithium users, and both users compared with the matched non-user controls. Patients who were prescribed only valproate or both valproate and lithium showed a 56% or 62% increased risk of dementia, respectively, than those who were not prescribed both medications. However, lithium-only users did not show a significant increase in the risk of dementia, so that lithium has the potential to be a relatively safer choice than valproate when considering the risk of dementia in OABD patients [80].

An open study of lamotrigine add-on to lithium or valproic acid suggested antidepressant efficacy in geriatric BD patients [81]. A post hoc analysis of two studies confirmed that lamotrigine also prolonged time to a depressive relapse in patients ≥55 years [82].

Antipsychotics are a first-line treatment in acute mania, yet their usage in geriatric patients needs a careful clinical evaluation due to the increased mortality for cardio- and cerebrovascular events, at least in patients with dementia (FDA Black box warning from 2005) [83]. Second-generation antipsychotics (SGA) are commonly used and proved to be beneficial concerning mood-stabilizing effects [84]. For acute mania, post hoc evidence from a controlled study exists for quetiapine, and open label trials and case series suggest also efficacy for asenapine, aripiprazole, clozapine, and risperidone [40]. Studies of SGA in bipolar depression and maintenance in old age BD, however, are lacking.

Antidepressants can provide short-term benefit, with known increased risk of mania and rapid cycling in long term in BD-I patients with relevant risk factors [84]. On the other hand, the natural odds of a manic recurrence also decrease with age. So that the choice whether continue an antidepressant treatment or not should be built on a case-to-case basis [40].

Electroconvulsive therapy (ECT) constitutes an alternative treatment modality to treat both mania and depression [86] and can also be used in continuation treatment [87]. Despite an overall lack of robust evidence both in OABD and BD in general, some studies demonstrated that not only mood, but also cognitive symptoms may improve with ECT, mediated by improvements in focus and depressive mood symptoms [88].

2.7 Conclusions

OABD is generally viewed as a special population within the bipolar disorder diagnosis which exhibits different characteristics compared to younger and middle-age BD patients. Specifically, despite an overall blunting of acute and severe BD symptoms, other manifestations become more severe, such as an increase in somatic comorbidities and cognitive impairment. The evolution of cognitive performance in OABD is not yet fully understood, apparently suggesting heterogeneous trajectories which underpin differential functional outcomes. Due to the different illness clinical presentation, as well as the unique therapeutic challenges that OABD presents, age should be taken into consideration in the clinical and research approaches, especially considering the progressive aging of the clinical, reflecting the general, populations.

References

1. Merikangas KR, Jin R, He J-P, Kessler RC, Lee S, Sampson NA, Viana MC, Andrade LH, Hu C, Karam EG, Ladea M, Medina-Mora ME, Ono Y, Posada-Villa J, Sagar R, Wells JE, Zarkov Z. Prevalence and correlates of bipolar spectrum disorder in the world mental health survey initiative. Arch Gen Psychiatry. 2011;68:241–51. https://doi.org/10.1001/archgenpsychiatry.2011.12.
2. Goetz I, Tohen M, Reed C, Lorenzo M, Vieta E, EMBLEM Advisory Board. Functional impairment in patients with mania: baseline results of the EMBLEM study. Bipolar Disord. 2007;9:45–52. https://doi.org/10.1111/j.1399-5618.2007.00325.x.
3. Rosa AR, Franco C, Martínez-Aran A, Sánchez-Moreno J, Reinares M, Salamero M, Arango C, Ayuso-Mateos JL, Kapczinski F, Vieta E. Functional impairment in patients with remitted bipolar disorder. Psychother Psychosom. 2008;77:390–2. https://doi.org/10.1159/000151520.
4. Strakowski SM, Williams JR, Fleck DE, Delbello MP. Eight-month functional outcome from mania following a first psychiatric hospitalization. J Psychiatr Res. 2000;34:193–200. https://doi.org/10.1016/s0022-3956(00)00015-7.
5. IsHak WW, Brown K, Aye SS, Kahloon M, Mobaraki S, Hanna R. Health-related quality of life in bipolar disorder. Bipolar Disord. 2012;14:6–18. https://doi.org/10.1111/j.1399-5618.2011.00969.x.
6. Michalak EE, Yatham LN, Lam RW. Quality of life in bipolar disorder: a review of the literature. Health Qual Life Outcomes. 2005;3:72. https://doi.org/10.1186/1477-7525-3-72.
7. Ferrari AJ, Stockings E, Khoo J-P, Erskine HE, Degenhardt L, Vos T, Whiteford HA. The prevalence and burden of bipolar disorder: findings from the Global Burden of Disease Study 2013. Bipolar Disord. 2016;18:440–50. https://doi.org/10.1111/bdi.12423.
8. Bonnín CM, Sánchez-Moreno J, Martínez-Arán A, Solé B, Reinares M, Rosa AR, Goikolea JM, Benabarre A, Ayuso-Mateos JL, Ferrer M, Vieta E, Torrent C. Subthreshold symptoms in bipolar disorder: impact on neurocognition, quality of life and disability. J Affect Disord. 2012;136:650–9. https://doi.org/10.1016/j.jad.2011.10.012.
9. Hirschfeld RMA, Calabrese JR, Weissman MM, Reed M, Davies MA, Frye MA, Keck PE, Lewis L, McElroy SL, McNulty JP, Wagner KD. Screening for bipolar disorder in the community. J Clin Psychiatry. 2003;64:53–9. https://doi.org/10.4088/jcp.v64n0111.
10. Depp CA, Jeste DV. Bipolar disorder in older adults: a critical review. Bipolar Disord. 2004;6:343–67. https://doi.org/10.1111/j.1399-5618.2004.00139.x.
11. Jeste DV, Alexopoulos GS, Bartels SJ, Cummings JL, Gallo JJ, Gottlieb GL, Halpain MC, Palmer BW, Patterson TL, Reynolds CF, Lebowitz BD. Consensus statement on the upcoming crisis in geriatric mental. Research agenda for the next 2 decades. Arch Gen Psychiatry. 1999; https://doi.org/10.1001/archpsyc.56.9.848.
12. Sajatovic M, Strejilevich SA, Gildengers AG, Dols A, Al Jurdi RK, Forester BP, Kessing LV, Beyer J, Manes F, Rej S, Rosa AR, Schouws SNTM, Tsai SY, Young RC, Shulman KI. A report on older-age bipolar disorder from the International Society for Bipolar Disorders Task Force. Bipolar Disord. 2015; https://doi.org/10.1111/bdi.12331.
13. Oostervink F, Boomsma MM, Nolen WA, Advisory Board EMBLEM. Bipolar disorder in the elderly; different effects of age and of age of onset. J Affect Disord. 2009;116:176–83. https://doi.org/10.1016/j.jad.2008.11.012.
14. Dols A, Beekman A. Older age bipolar disorder. Psychiatr Clin N Am. 2018; https://doi.org/10.1016/j.psc.2017.10.008.
15. Sajatovic M, Dols A, Rej S, Almeida OP, Beunders AJM, Blumberg HP, Briggs FBS, Forester BP, Patrick RE, Forlenza OV, Gildengers A, Jimenez E, Vieta E, Mulsant B, Schouws S, Paans N, Strejilevich S, Sutherland A, Tsai S, Wilson B, Eyler LT. Bipolar symptoms, somatic burden, and functioning in older-age bipolar disorder: analyses from the Global Aging & Geriatric Experiments in Bipolar Disorder Database project. Bipolar Disord. 2021;1–12 https://doi.org/10.1111/bdi.13119.

16. Kessing LV. Diagnostic subtypes of bipolar disorder in older versus younger adults. Bipolar Disord. 2006;8:56–64. https://doi.org/10.1111/j.1399-5618.2006.00278.x.
17. Nivoli AMA, Murru A, Pacchiarotti I, Valenti M, Rosa AR, Hidalgo D, Virdis V, Strejilevich S, Vieta E, Colom F. Bipolar disorder in the elderly: a cohort study comparing older and younger patients. Acta Psychiatr Scand. 2014;130:364–73. https://doi.org/10.1111/acps.12272.
18. Kessing LV, Hansen MG, Andersen PK. Course of illness in depressive and bipolar disorders. Naturalistic study, 1994-1999. Br J Psychiatry. 2004;185:372–7. https://doi.org/10.1192/bjp.185.5.372.
19. Kessing LV. Recurrence in affective disorder. II. Effect of age and gender. Br J Psychiatry. 1998;172:29–34. https://doi.org/10.1192/bjp.172.1.29.
20. Sajatovic M, Blow FC, Ignacio RV, Kales HC. Age-related modifiers of clinical presentation and health service use among veterans with bipolar disorder. Psychiatr Serv. 2004;55:1014–21. https://doi.org/10.1176/appi.ps.55.9.1014.
21. Depp CA, Lindamer LA, Folsom DP, Gilmer T, Hough RL, Garcia P, Jeste DV. Differences in clinical features and mental health service use in bipolar disorder across the lifespan. Am J Geriatr Psychiatry. 2005;13:290–8. https://doi.org/10.1176/appi.ajgp.13.4.290.
22. Schürhoff F, Bellivier F, Jouvent R, Mouren-Siméoni MC, Bouvard M, Allilaire JF, Leboyer M. Early and late onset bipolar disorders: two different forms of manic-depressive illness? J Affect Disord. 2000;58:215–21. https://doi.org/10.1016/s0165-0327(99)00111-1.
23. Eyler LT, Briggs FBS, Dols A, Rej S, Almeida OP, Beunders AJM, Blumberg HP, Forester BP, Patrick RE, Forlenza OV, Gildengers A, Jimenez E, Vieta E, Mulsant BH, Schouws S, Paans NPG, Strejilevich S, Sutherland A, Tsai S, Sajatovic M. Symptom severity mixity in older-age bipolar bisorder: analyses from the global aging and geriatric experiments in bipolar disorder database (GAGE-BD). Am J Geriatr Psychiatry. 2022; https://doi.org/10.1016/j.jagp.2022.03.007.
24. Orhan M, Korten N, Stek M, Comijs H, Schouws S, Dols A. The relationship between cognitive and social functioning in older patients with bipolar disorder. J Affect Disord. 2018;240:177–82. https://doi.org/10.1016/j.jad.2018.07.055.
25. Beunders AJM, Klaus F, Kok AAL, Schouws SNTM, Kupka RW, Blumberg HP, Briggs F, Eyler LT, Forester BP, Forlenza OV, Gildengers A, Jimenez E, Mulsant BH, Patrick RE, Rej S, Sajatovic M, Sarna K, Sutherland A, Yala J, Vieta E, Villa LM, Korten NCM, Dols A. Bipolar I and bipolar II subtypes in older age: results from the Global Aging and Geriatric Experiments in Bipolar Disorder (GAGE-BD) project. Bipolar Disord. 2022;00:17. https://doi.org/10.1111/BDI.13271.
26. Miller JN, Black DW. Bipolar disorder and suicide: a review. Curr Psychiatry Rep. 2020;22:6. https://doi.org/10.1007/s11920-020-1130-0.
27. Schaffer A, Isometsä ET, Azorin J-M, Cassidy F, Goldstein T, Rihmer Z, Sinyor M, Tondo L, Moreno DH, Turecki G, Reis C, Kessing LV, Ha K, Weizman A, Beautrais A, Chou Y-H, Diazgranados N, Levitt AJ, Zarate CA, Yatham L. A review of factors associated with greater likelihood of suicide attempts and suicide deaths in bipolar disorder: Part II of a report of the International Society for Bipolar Disorders Task Force on Suicide in Bipolar Disorder. Aust N Z J Psychiatry. 2015;49:1006–20. https://doi.org/10.1177/0004867415594428.
28. Aizenberg D, Olmer A, Barak Y. Suicide attempts amongst elderly bipolar patients. J Affect Disord. 2006;91:91–4. https://doi.org/10.1016/j.jad.2005.12.013.
29. Fries GR, Zamzow MJ, Andrews T, Pink O, Scaini G, Quevedo J. Accelerated aging in bipolar disorder: a comprehensive review of molecular findings and their clinical implications. Neurosci Biobehav Rev. 2020;112:107–16. https://doi.org/10.1016/J.NEUBIOREV.2020.01.035.
30. Lima CNC, Suchting R, Scaini G, Cuellar VA, Del Favero-Campbell A, Walss-Bass C, Soares JC, Quevedo J, Fries GR. Epigenetic GrimAge acceleration and cognitive impairment in bipolar disorder. Eur Neuropsychopharmacol. 2022;62:10–21. https://doi.org/10.1016/J.EURONEURO.2022.06.007.
31. Abé C, Ching CRK, Liberg B, Lebedev AV, Agartz I, Akudjedu TN, Alda M, Alnæs D, Alonso-Lana S, Benedetti F, Berk M, Bøen E, Bonnin CDM, Breuer F, Brosch K, Brouwer RM, Canales-Rodríguez EJ, Cannon DM, Chye Y, Dahl A, Dandash O, Dannlowski U, Dohm

K, Elvsåshagen T, Fisch L, Fullerton JM, Goikolea JM, Grotegerd D, Haatveit B, Hahn T, Hajek T, Heindel W, Ingvar M, Sim K, Kircher TTJ, Lenroot RK, Malt UF, McDonald C, McWhinney SR, Melle I, Meller T, Melloni EMT, Mitchell PB, Nabulsi L, Nenadić I, Opel N, Overs BJ, Panicalli F, Pfarr JK, Poletti S, Pomarol-Clotet E, Radua J, Repple J, Ringwald KG, Roberts G, Rodriguez-Cano E, Salvador R, Sarink K, Sarró S, Schmitt S, Stein F, Suo C, Thomopoulos SI, Tronchin G, Vieta E, Westlye LT, White AG, Yatham LN, Zak N, Thompson PM, Andreassen OA, Landén M. Longitudinal structural brain changes in bipolar disorder: a Multicenter Neuroimaging Study of 1232 Individuals by the ENIGMA Bipolar Disorder Working Group. Biol Psychiatry. 2021; https://doi.org/10.1016/j.biopsych.2021.09.008.

32. Lala SV, Sajatovic M. Medical and psychiatric comorbidities among elderly individuals with bipolar disorder: a literature review. J Geriatr Psychiatry Neurol. 2012; https://doi.org/10.1177/0891988712436683.
33. Dols A, Beekman A. Older age bipolar disorder. Clin Geriatr Med. 2020; https://doi.org/10.1016/j.cger.2019.11.008.
34. Rise IV, Haro JM, Gjervan B. Clinical features, comorbidity, and cognitive impairment in elderly bipolar patients. Neuropsychiatr Dis Treat. 2016; https://doi.org/10.2147/NDT.S100843.
35. Tsai S-Y, Kuo C-J, Chung K-H, Huang Y-L, Lee H-C, Chen C-C. Cognitive dysfunction and medical morbidity in elderly outpatients with bipolar disorder. Am J Geriatr Psychiatry. 2009;17:1004–11. https://doi.org/10.1097/JGP.0b013e3181b7ef2a.
36. Almeida OP, Dols A, Blanken MAJT, Rej S, Blumberg HP, Villa L, Forester BP, Forlenza OV, Gildengers A, Vieta E, Jimenez E, Mulsant B, Schouws S, Tsai S, Korten NCM, Sutherland A, Briggs FBS, Flicker L, Eyler LT, Sajatovic M. Physical health burden among older men and women with bipolar disorder: results from the gage-bd collaboration. Am J Geriatr Psychiatr. 2022;30:727–32. https://doi.org/10.1016/j.jagp.2021.12.006.
37. Beunders AJM, Kok AAL, Kosmas PC, Beekman ATF, Sonnenberg CM, Schouws SNTM, Kupka RW, Stek ML, Dols A. Physical comorbidity in Older-Age Bipolar Disorder (OABD) compared to the general population—a 3-year longitudinal prospective cohort study. J Affect Disord. 2021;288:83–91. https://doi.org/10.1016/j.jad.2021.03.057.
38. Bauer IE, Gálvez JF, Hamilton JE, Balanzá-Martínez V, Zunta-Soares GB, Soares JC, Meyer TD. Lifestyle interventions targeting dietary habits and exercise in bipolar disorder: a systematic review. J Psychiatr Res. 2016;74:1–7. https://doi.org/10.1016/j.jpsychires.2015.12.006.
39. Dols A, Rhebergen D, Beekman A, Kupka R, Sajatovic M, Stek ML. Psychiatric and medical comorbidities: results from a bipolar elderly cohort study. Am J Geriatr Psychiatr. 2014;22:1066–74. https://doi.org/10.1016/j.jagp.2013.12.176.
40. Ljubic N, Ueberberg B, Grunze H, Assion HJ. Treatment of bipolar disorders in older adults: a review. Ann General Psychiatry. 2021;20:1–11. https://doi.org/10.1186/s12991-021-00367-x.
41. Depp CA, Jin H, Mohamed S, Kaskow J, Moore DJ, Jeste DV. Bipolar disorder in middle-aged and elderly adults: is age of onset important? J Nerv Ment Dis. 2004;192:796–9. https://doi.org/10.1097/01.nmd.0000145055.45944.d6.
42. Ramírez-Bermúdez J, Marrufo-Melendez O, Berlanga-Flores C, Guadamuz A, Atriano C, Carrillo-Mezo R, Alvarado P, Favila R, Taboada J, Rios C, Yoldi-Negrete M, Ruiz-Garcia R, Tohen M. White matter abnormalities in late onset first episode mania: a diffusion tensor imaging study. Am J Geriatr Psychiatry. 2021; https://doi.org/10.1016/j.jagp.2021.03.007.
43. Subramaniam H, Dennis MS, Byrne EJ. The role of vascular risk factors in late onset bipolar disorder. Int J Geriatr Psychiatry. 2007;22:733–7. https://doi.org/10.1002/gps.1730.
44. Schouws SNTM, Stek ML, Comijs HC, Beekman ATF. Risk factors for cognitive impairment in elderly bipolar patients. J Affect Disord. 2010;125:330–5. https://doi.org/10.1016/j.jad.2009.12.004.
45. Vasudev A, Thomas A. "Bipolar disorder" in the elderly: what's in a name? Maturitas. 2010;66:231–5. https://doi.org/10.1016/j.maturitas.2010.02.013.
46. Schouws SNTM, Comijs HC, Stek ML, Dekker J, Oostervink F, Naarding P, Van Der Velde I, Beekman ATF. Cognitive impairment in early and late bipolar disorder. Am J Geriatr Psychiatr. 2009;17:508–15. https://doi.org/10.1097/JGP.0b013e31819e2d50.

47. Lavin P, Buck G, Almeida OP, Su C-L, Eyler LT, Dols A, Blumberg HP, Forester BP, Forlenza OV, Gildengers A, Mulsant BH, Tsai S-Y, Vieta E, Schouws S, Briggs FBS, Sutherland A, Sarna K, Yala J, Orhan M, Korten N, Sajatovic M, Rej S. Clinical correlates of late-onset versus early-onset bipolar disorder in a global sample of older adults. Int J Geriatr Psychiatry. 2022;37 https://doi.org/10.1002/GPS.5833.
48. Bourne C, Aydemir O, Balanzá-Martínez V, Bora E, Brissos S, Cavanagh JTO, Clark L, Cubukcuoglu Z, Dias VV, Dittmann S, Ferrier IN, Fleck DE, Frangou S, Gallagher P, Jones L, Kieseppä T, Martínez-Aran A, Melle I, Moore PB, Mur M, Pfennig A, Raust A, Senturk V, Simonsen C, Smith DJ, Bio DS, Soeiro-de-Souza MG, Stoddart SDR, Sundet K, Szöke A, Thompson JM, Torrent C, Zalla T, Craddock N, Andreassen OA, Leboyer M, Vieta E, Bauer M, Worhunsky PD, Tzagarakis C, Rogers RD, Geddes JR, Goodwin GM. Neuropsychological testing of cognitive impairment in euthymic bipolar disorder: an individual patient data meta-analysis. Acta Psychiatr Scand. 2013;128:149–62. https://doi.org/10.1111/acps.12133.
49. Mann-Wrobel MC, Carreno JT, Dickinson D. Meta-analysis of neuropsychological functioning in euthymic bipolar disorder: an update and investigation of moderator variables. Bipolar Disord. 2011;13:334–42. https://doi.org/10.1111/j.1399-5618.2011.00935.x.
50. Torres IJ, Boudreau VG, Yatham LN. Neuropsychological functioning in euthymic bipolar disorder: a meta-analysis. Acta Psychiatr Scand. 2007;116:17–26. https://doi.org/10.1111/j.1600-0447.2007.01055.x.
51. Montejo L, Torrent C, Jiménez E, Martínez-Arán A, Blumberg HP, Burdick KE, Chen P, Dols A, Eyler LT, Forester BP, Gatchel JR, Gildengers A, Kessing LV, Miskowiak KW, Olagunju AT, Patrick RE, Schouws S, Radua J, Bonnín CDM, Vieta E. Cognition in older adults with bipolar disorder: an ISBD task force systematic review and meta-analysis based on a comprehensive neuropsychological assessment. Bipolar Disord. 2022;24:115–36. https://doi.org/10.1111/bdi.13175.
52. Montejo L, Jiménez E, Torrent C, Bonnín CDM, Solé B, Martínez-Arán A, Vieta E, Moreno JS. Functional Remediation for Older Adults with Bipolar Disorder (FROA-BD): study protocol for a randomized controlled trial. Rev Psiquiatr Salud Ment. 2022; https://doi.org/10.1016/j.rpsm.2022.01.004.
53. Cardoso T, Bauer IE, Meyer TD, Kapczinski F, Soares JC. Neuroprogression and cognitive functioning in bipolar disorder: a systematic review. Curr Psychiatry Rep. 2015;17:75. https://doi.org/10.1007/s11920-015-0605-x.
54. Kapczinski NS, Mwangi B, Cassidy RM, Librenza-Garcia D, Bermudez MB, Kauer-Sant'anna M, Kapczinski F, Passos IC. Neuroprogression and illness trajectories in bipolar disorder. Expert Rev Neurother. 2017; https://doi.org/10.1080/14737175.2017.1240615.
55. Salagre E, Dodd S, Aedo A, Rosa A, Amoretti S, Pinzon J, Reinares M, Berk M, Kapczinski FP, Vieta E, Grande I. Toward precision psychiatry in bipolar disorder: staging 2.0. front. Psychiatry. 2018;9:641.
56. Berk M, Kapczinski F, Andreazza AC, Dean OM, Giorlando F, Maes M, Yücel M, Gama CS, Dodd S, Dean B, Magalhães PVS, Amminger P, McGorry P, Malhi GS. Pathways underlying neuroprogression in bipolar disorder: focus on inflammation, oxidative stress and neurotrophic factors. Neurosci Biobehav Rev. 2011; https://doi.org/10.1016/j.neubiorev.2010.10.001.
57. Millett CE, Burdick KE. Defining heterogeneous cognitive trajectories in bipolar disorder: a perspective. Harv Rev Psychiatry. 2021; https://doi.org/10.1097/HRP.0000000000000297.
58. Passos IC, Mwangi B, Vieta E, Berk M, Kapczinski F. Areas of controversy in neuroprogression in bipolar disorder. Acta Psychiatr Scand. 2016; https://doi.org/10.1111/acps.12581.
59. Delaloye C, Moy G, De Bilbao F, Weber K, Baudois S, Haller S, Xekardaki A, Canuto A, Giardini U, Lövblad KO, Gold G, Giannakopoulos P. Longitudinal analysis of cognitive performances and structural brain changes in late-life bipolar disorder. Int J Geriatr Psychiatry. 2011;26:1309–18. https://doi.org/10.1002/gps.2683.
60. Schouws S, Comijs HC, Dols A, Beekman ATF, Stek ML. Five-year follow-up of cognitive impairment in older adults with bipolar disorder. Bipolar Disord. 2016;18:148–54. https://doi.org/10.1111/bdi.12374.

61. Szmulewicz A, Valerio MP, Martino DJ. Longitudinal analysis of cognitive performances in recent-onset and late-life bipolar disorder: a systematic review and meta-analysis. Bipolar Disord. 2019; https://doi.org/10.1111/bdi.12841.
62. Gildengers AG, Mulsant BH, Begley A, Mazumdar S, Hyams AV, Reynolds CF, Kupfer DJ, Butters MA. The longitudinal course of cognition in older adults with bipolar disorder. Bipolar Disord. 2009;11:744–52. https://doi.org/10.1111/j.1399-5618.2009.00739.x.
63. Lewandowski KE, Sperry SH, Malloy MC, Forester BP. Age as a predictor of cognitive decline in bipolar disorder. Am J Geriatr Psychiatry. 2014;22:1462–8. https://doi.org/10.1016/j.jagp.2013.10.002.
64. Seelye A, Thuras P, Doane B, Clason C, VanVoorst W, Urošević S. Steeper aging-related declines in cognitive control processes among adults with bipolar disorders. J Affect Disord. 2019;246:595–602. https://doi.org/10.1016/j.jad.2018.12.076.
65. Montejo L, Solé B, Jiménez E, Borràs R, Clougher D, Reinares M, Portella MJ, Martinez-Aran A, Vieta E, Del Mar Bonnín C, Torrent C. Aging in bipolar disorder: cognitive performance and clinical factors based on an adulthood-lifespan perspective. J Affect Disord. 2022;312:292–302. https://doi.org/10.1016/j.jad.2022.06.030.
66. Da Silva J, Gonçalves-Pereira M, Xavier M, Mukaetova-Ladinska EB. Affective disorders and risk of developing dementia: systematic review. Br J Psychiatry. 2013; https://doi.org/10.1192/bjp.bp.111.101931.
67. Velosa J, Delgado A, Finger E, Berk M, Kapczinski F, de Azevedo Cardoso T. Risk of dementia in bipolar disorder and the interplay of lithium: a systematic review and meta-analyses. Acta Psychiatr Scand. 2020; https://doi.org/10.1111/acps.13153.
68. Wu KY, Chang CM, Liang HY, Wu CS, Chia-Hsuan W, Chia-Hsuan Wu E, Chau YL, Tsai HJ. Increased risk of developing dementia in patients with bipolar disorder: a nested matched case-control study. Bipolar Disord. 2013;15:787–94. https://doi.org/10.1111/bdi.12116.
69. Kessing LV, Andersen PK. Does the risk of developing dementia increase with the number of episodes in patients with depressive disorder and in patients with bipolar disorder? J Neurol Neurosurg Psychiatry. 2004;75:1662–6. https://doi.org/10.1136/jnnp.2003.031773.
70. Forlenza OV, Aprahamian I. Cognitive impairment and dementia in bipolar disorder. Front Biosci (Elite Ed). 2013;5:258–65.
71. Forlenza OV, Aprahamian I, Radanovic M, Talib LL, Camargo MZA, Stella F, Machado-Vieira R, Gattaz WF. Cognitive impairment in late-life bipolar disorder is not associated with Alzheimer's disease pathological signature in the cerebrospinal fluid. Bipolar Disord. 2016;18:63–70. https://doi.org/10.1111/bdi.12360.
72. Baez S, Pinasco C, Roca M, Ferrari J, Couto B, García-Cordero I, Ibañez A, Cruz F, Reyes P, Matallana D, Manes F, Cetcovich M, Torralva T. Brain structural correlates of executive and social cognition profiles in behavioral variant frontotemporal dementia and elderly bipolar disorder. Neuropsychologia. 2019;126:159–69. https://doi.org/10.1016/j.neuropsychologia.2017.02.012. Epub 2017 Feb 17. PMID: 28219620.
73. Ducharme S, Dols A, Laforce R, Devenney E, Kumfor F, Van Den Stock J, Dallaire-Théroux C, Seelaar H, Gossink F, Vijverberg E, Huey E, Vandenbulcke M, Masellis M, Trieu C, Onyike C, Caramelli P, De Souza LC, Santillo A, Waldö ML, Landin-Romero R, Piguet O, Kelso W, Eratne D, Velakoulis D, Ikeda M, Perry D, Pressman P, Boeve B, Vandenberghe R, Mendez M, Azuar C, Levy R, Le Ber I, Baez S, Lerner A, Ellajosyula R, Pasquier F, Galimberti D, Scarpini E, Van Swieten J, Hornberger M, Rosen H, Hodges J, Diehl-Schmid J, Pijnenburg Y. Recommendations to distinguish behavioural variant frontotemporal dementia from psychiatric disorders. Brain. 2020;143:1632. https://doi.org/10.1093/BRAIN/AWAA018.
74. Lotrich FE, Pollock BG. Aging and clinical pharmacology: implications for antidepressants. J Clin Pharmacol. 2005;45:1106–22. https://doi.org/10.1177/0091270005280297.
75. Shulman KI, Almeida OP, Herrmann N, Schaffer A, Strejilevich SA, Paternoster C, Amodeo S, Dols A, Sajatovic M. Delphi survey of maintenance lithium treatment in older adults with bipolar disorder: an ISBD task force report. Bipolar Disord. 2019;21:117–23. https://doi.org/10.1111/BDI.12714.

76. Young RC, Mulsant BH, Sajatovic M, Gildengers AG, Gyulai L, Al Jurdi RK, Beyer J, Evans J, Banerjee S, Greenberg R, Marino P, Kunik ME, Chen P, Barrett M, Schulberg HC, Bruce ML, Reynolds CIF, Alexopoulos GS. GERI-BD: a randomized double-blind controlled trial of lithium and divalproex in the treatment of mania in older patients with bipolar disorder. Am J Psychiatry. 2017;174:1086–93. https://doi.org/10.1176/APPI.AJP.2017.15050657.
77. Schoretsanitis G, de Filippis R, Brady BM, Homan P, Suppes T, Kane JM. Prevalence of impaired kidney function in patients with long-term lithium treatment: a systematic review and meta-analysis. Bipolar Disord. 2022;24:264–74. https://doi.org/10.1111/BDI.13154.
78. Tondo L, Abramowicz M, Alda M, Bauer M, Bocchetta A, Bolzani L, Calkin CV, Chillotti C, Hidalgo-Mazzei D, Manchia M, Müller-Oerlinghausen B, Murru A, Perugi G, Pinna M, Quaranta G, Reginaldi D, Reif A, Ritter P, Rybakowski JK, Saiger D, Sani G, Selle V, Stamm T, Vázquez GH, Veeh J, Vieta E, Baldessarini RJ. Long-term lithium treatment in bipolar disorder: effects on glomerular filtration rate and other metabolic parameters. Int J Bipolar Disord. 2017;5 https://doi.org/10.1186/S40345-017-0096-2.
79. Yatham LN, Chakrabarty T, Bond DJ, Schaffer A, Beaulieu S, Parikh SV, McIntyre RS, Milev RV, Alda M, Vazquez G, Ravindran AV, Frey BN, Sharma V, Goldstein BI, Rej S, O'Donovan C, Tourjman V, Kozicky JM, Kauer-Sant'Anna M, Malhi G, Suppes T, Vieta E, Kapczinski F, Kanba S, Lam RW, Kennedy SH, Calabrese J, Berk M, Post R. Canadian Network for Mood and Anxiety Treatments (CANMAT) and International Society for Bipolar Disorders (ISBD) recommendations for the management of patients with bipolar disorder with mixed presentations. Bipolar Disord. 2021;23:767–88. https://doi.org/10.1111/BDI.13135.
80. Moon W, Ji E, Shin J, Kwon JS, Kim KW. Effect of valproate and lithium on dementia onset risk in bipolar disorder patients. Sci Rep. 2022;12 https://doi.org/10.1038/S41598-022-18350-1.
81. Robillard M, Conn DK. Lamotrigine use in geriatric patients with bipolar depression. Can J Psychiatr. 2002;47:767–70. https://doi.org/10.1177/070674370204700808.
82. Sajatovic M, Gyulai L, Calabrese JR, Thompson TR, Wilson B, White R, Evoniuk G. Maintenance treatment outcomes in older patients with bipolar I disorder. Am J Geriatr Psychiatry. 2005;13:305–11. https://doi.org/10.1176/APPI.AJGP.13.4.305.
83. Jeste DV, Blazer D, Casey D, Meeks T, Salzman C, Schneider L, Tariot P, Yaffe K. ACNP White Paper: update on use of antipsychotic drugs in elderly persons with dementia. Neuropsychopharmacology. 2008;33:957–70. https://doi.org/10.1038/SJ.NPP.1301492.
84. Goodwin GM, Haddad PM, Ferrier IN, Aronson JK, Barnes TRH, Cipriani A, Coghill DR, Fazel S, Geddes JR, Grunze H, Holmes EA, Howes O, Hudson S, Hunt N, Jones I, MacMillan IC, McAllister-Williams H, Miklowitz DR, Morriss R, Munafò M, Paton C, Saharkian BJ, Saunders KEA, Sinclair JMA, Taylor D, Vieta E, Young AH. Evidence-based guidelines for treating bipolar disorder: revised third edition recommendations from the British Association for Psychopharmacology. J Psychopharmacol. 2016;30:495–553. https://doi.org/10.1177/0269881116636545.
85. Takano C, Kato M, Adachi N, Kubota Y, Azekawa T, Ueda H, Edagawa K, Katsumoto E, Goto E, Hongo S, Miki K, Tsuboi T, Yasui-Furukori N, Nakagawa A, Kikuchi T, Watanabe K, Kinoshita T, Yoshimura R. Clinical characteristics and prescriptions associated with a 2-year course of rapid cycling and euthymia in bipolar disorder: a multicenter treatment survey for bipolar disorder in psychiatric clinics. Front Psych. 2023;14 https://doi.org/10.3389/FPSYT.2023.1183782.
86. Versiani M, Cheniaux E, Landeira-Fernandez J. Efficacy and safety of electroconvulsive therapy in the treatment of bipolar disorder: a systematic review. J ECT. 2011;27:153–64. https://doi.org/10.1097/YCT.0B013E3181E6332E.
87. Hausmann A, Post T, Post F, Dehning J, Kemmler G, Grunze H. Efficacy of continuation/maintenance electroconvulsive therapy in the treatment of patients with mood disorders: a retrospective analysis. J ECT. 2019;35:122–6. https://doi.org/10.1097/YCT.0000000000000547.
88. Tielkes CEM, Comijs HC, Verwijk E, Stek ML. The effects of ECT on cognitive functioning in the elderly: a review. Int J Geriatr Psychiatry. 2008;23:789–95. https://doi.org/10.1002/GPS.1989.

Alcohol Abuse and Addiction in Older People

3

Dorota Religa, Theofanis Tsevis, and Lars-Olof Wahlund

3.1 Epidemiology of Alcohol Abuse in the Older Population

3.1.1 Introduction

There is evidence to suggest that alcohol abuse in older people has increased over the last few decades, particularly in developed countries with aging populations [1, 2]. Several studies have documented a rising trend in alcohol consumption among older adults, with some studies indicating that rates of alcohol overconsumption among older individuals have doubled in the past decade [3]. Several factors may be contributing to this trend, including changes in social attitudes toward alcohol use, increasing rates of stress and anxiety among older adults, and the growing availability and affordability of alcohol. In addition, the aging process itself can influence older people's grade of susceptibility to conditions associated with alcohol overconsumption [4].

One factor that may be contributing to the increase in alcohol abuse among older individuals is the "baby boomer" generation, which is now entering their senior years. This generation has historically had increased proportion of alcohol and drug abuse than previous generations, and they may be continuing these patterns of behavior into their later years [5]. According to epidemiological data, as the generation of baby boomers approach the retirement stage, older individuals are estimated to outnumber the children population within the next 10 years. That fact poses great challenges in front of healthcare and health policy strategies. Alcohol abuse and addiction in older individuals, although it corresponds to the most common substance abuse, are not sufficiently reported and thus underdiagnosed. It is, moreover,

D. Religa · T. Tsevis (✉) · L.-O. Wahlund
Department of Neurobiology, Care Sciences and Society; Division of Clinical Geriatrics, Karolinska Institutet, Stockholm, Sweden
e-mail: Dorota.Religa@ki.se; Theofanis.Tsevis@ki.se; Lars-Olof.Wahlund@ki.se

N. Veronese, A. Marseglia (eds.), *Psychogeriatrics*, Practical Issues in Geriatrics,
https://doi.org/10.1007/978-3-031-58488-6_3

noticed that a greater proportion of female older individuals has developed tendency to episodic drinking and alcohol abuse during the last decades [6].

There are two groups: The first one consists of individuals, having developed alcohol abuse earlier than 65 years of age. They represent the two-thirds of all individuals above 65 years, are mostly men, with higher burden of somatic and psychiatric comorbidities. Almost one-third of individuals older than 65 years has developed alcohol abuse in late life. They have milder profile of alcohol disorders, and the proportion of women is greater. Alcohol consumption is usually related to stressful events and loneliness [1].

The prevalence of alcohol overconsumption among older individuals varies depending on the definition used, but estimates suggest that 4% of older adults have alcohol use disorder (AUD) [7]. Moreover, there is a higher proportion, at least 10%, of older adults having experienced binge drinking during the last month [3]. Men are more likely to engage in heavy drinking and alcohol abuse compared to women in the elderly population. The prevalence of alcohol abuse decreases with age, with those aged 75 and older having a decreased risk of alcohol abuse compared to those aged 65–74. Alcohol abuse is often associated with other medical and psychiatric comorbidities, such as depression, anxiety, cognitive impairment, and liver disease, among others. Alcohol abuse among older people is related to a higher mortality risk due to both acute and chronic health conditions. Elderly individuals with alcohol abuse disorders may be less likely to seek treatment compared to younger individuals [4].

Prevalence varies also across different countries and continents. It is a significant public health concern in many European countries, for example, in the UK, alcohol-related hospital admissions among those aged 65 and older have increased in recent years [8, 9]. In the US, alcohol abuse is more common among younger age-groups, but the prevalence among older people is increasing [10]. In Canada, alcohol abuse is also a growing concern among the elderly population [11]. Alcohol abuse in populations of older individuals is a growing concern in many Asian countries, such as China, Japan, and Korea [12]. The prevalence of alcohol abuse is often increased among men compared to women in these countries. There is limited research on alcohol abuse in the elderly population in Africa. However, studies suggest that alcohol abuse is a significant concern among elderly individuals in some African countries, such as South Africa [13]. In many South American countries, alcohol overconsumption is an important public health concern, but there is limited research on alcohol abuse among the elderly population. Finally, alcohol abuse among older adults varies across different countries and continents, and healthcare providers should be aware of the cultural, social, and economic factors that influence alcohol use among this population. It is important to develop tailored interventions and treatment plans for elderly individuals struggling with alcohol abuse that take into account the unique cultural and social contexts in which they live. In conclusion, alcohol abuse is a significant public health concern among the elderly population, and its prevalence is increasing worldwide. Healthcare providers should be aware of the epidemiological factors associated with alcohol overconsumption among older individuals and take steps to identify and address alcohol abuse in this vulnerable population.

3.1.2 Environmental and Genetic Factors

Cultural characteristics across different countries and continents can affect alcohol consumption in the elderly population. Cultural attitudes toward alcohol can vary widely, with some cultures having a more permissive attitude toward alcohol use than others. For example, in some cultures, drinking alcohol is an accepted part of socializing and celebrations, while in others, it is considered taboo. Elderly individuals who belong to cultures that value family and community may be at risk of alcohol abuse if they experience social isolation. This can be due to a lack of social support, limited access to healthcare services, and other factors. Cultural attitudes toward alcoholism may lead to stigma and shame for elderly individuals who struggle with alcohol abuse. This can prevent them from seeking help and support. Religious beliefs can influence alcohol use in the elderly population. For example, some religions prohibit the consumption of alcohol, while others allow moderate alcohol use. Some cultures place a high value on aging gracefully and may view alcohol overconsumption among older individuals as a sign of weakness or moral failing. This can prevent elderly individuals from seeking help and support for alcohol abuse [14].

Socioeconomic status (SES) can also have an impact on alcohol abuse in the elderly population. According to the literature, alcohol consumption increases with higher SES [15]. However, older individuals with lower SES experiences significantly more negative alcohol-related consequences in comparison with those with higher status [16]. Those with lower SES may be more likely to experience social isolation and have limited social support, which can increase the harmful effect of alcohol abuse. Economic stress, such as financial strain and insecurity, can represent a risk factor for alcohol abuse in older individuals. They may have limited access to healthcare and substance abuse treatment services, such as counseling and medication-assisted treatment, which can make it more difficult to address alcohol abuse [17]. Regarding educational status, there is also a positive association between alcohol and educational level, but those having alcohol abuse have usually lower educational status [18]. Generally, older individuals with higher SES and educational status are characterized by light to moderate consumption, more frequent drinking, but lower proportion of binge drinking [19]. Elderly individuals with higher levels of education may have more knowledge about the risks of alcohol abuse and be more likely to engage in healthy behaviors. Moreover, they may have stronger social networks and better social support, as well as better job opportunities and economic stability, which can reduce stress and the risk of alcohol abuse [17].

Genetics can also play a role in alcohol abuse in the elderly population. Certain genetic variations have been related to higher risk of alcohol dependence, including variations in genes that affect the metabolism of alcohol, neurotransmitter systems, and stress response [20]. Elderly individuals with a family history of alcohol addiction or alcoholism may have a higher risk for alcohol-related problems [21]. Genetic factors may interact with environmental as well as socioeconomic factors, to pose a higher risk of alcohol overconsumption among older individuals [22]. Pharmacogenetic changes such as variations in genes that affect the metabolism of medications commonly prescribed to the elderly population, such as benzodiazepines and opioids, can also increase the risk of adverse reactions and interactions with alcohol [23].

3.1.3 Sex Differences in Alcohol Consumption

There are several sex differences in alcohol abuse among older people. While both men and women can experience alcohol-related problems as they age, there are different characteristics in the prevalence and consequences of alcohol intake. Men are more prone compared to women to consume alcohol and engage in heavy drinking [24]. However, the gender gap in alcohol use narrows as people age, and older women have higher risk of alcohol-related problems due to factors such as changes in metabolism and increased sensitivity to alcohol [25]. During the last decades, it noticed a relatively equal distribution of alcohol abuse in different age-groups in older men and women, related to higher grade of economic independence and socioeconomic status among women [26]. Generally, alcohol abuse including episodic alcohol intake in later life has been related to male gender, physical inactivity, burden of medications and particularly usage of anti-anxiety and sedative pills, and comorbidities including cognitive disorders [27].

Women are more likely than men to experience health complications related to alcohol use, for example, liver disease and cognitive impairment. This may be related to different physiological mechanisms in how alcohol is metabolized and how it affects the brain and other organs [25]. The effect of alcohol is more harmful among women than men, as the alcohol levels in blood are higher in women, when consuming the same amounts of alcohol with men. In addition, according to the literature, women seem to have higher pace of developing addiction and alcohol abuse and consequently they are more prone to alcohol-related diseases in liver or damages in the brain and the cardiovascular system [28]. There are a number of factors related to that difference, such as women's lower water content as well as lower body size, lower absorption rate related to higher fat levels and lower activity of alcohol dehydrogenase, which is an enzyme metabolizing alcohol [25]. Those factors act synergistically, leading to higher rate of alcohol passing through from the gastrointestinal system to the blood stream.

Social factors, such as gender-related roles and norms, can affect abuse among older adults. There are contradictory and mixed results in the literature regarding association between loneliness and adequate social interaction with alcohol, suggesting that geographical and cultural factors may influence that relationship [27]. Moreover, the fact that alcohol overconsumption among elderly is poorly mapped and underdiagnosed can be related to a change in beliefs regarding socially acceptable behaviors and attitudes. There is a relationship between high socioeconomic and educational status and high alcohol intake, even including women [26]. Those individuals are not being identified of primary care as they can hardly be suspected as alcohol abusers. Finally, the healthier an old person is the higher alcohol consumption has and by that means alcohol intake is regarding more as a health predictor, rather than the cause of diseases and health issues, and this seems to be more pronounced in women [27].

3.1.4 Drinking Levels

Standard drink has been selected as a tool of quantitative measurement of alcohol intake and corresponds to a beverage (beer, wine, liquor, or spirits), containing a certain amount of alcohol. It is used in guidelines created for addressing risks for health and in proposed recommendations for healthier lifestyles. This amount varies across different countries as there is no international agreement on specific alcohol levels. According to the World Health Organization, each standard drink should contain 10 g alcohol, but it ranges from 8 to 20 g around the world. In US, each standard drink contains 14 g alcohol [29].

As mentioned above, there are differences in the general population regarding the quantity of alcohol in each standard drink as well as diverse gender-specific recommendations regarding alcohol consumption across countries all over the world. Moderate drinking is defined as up to 2 standard drinks per day for men and as up to 1 standard drink per day for women. In addition, binge drinking, which corresponds to heavy episodic drinking within a short period of time, lasting at least 2 h and occurring at least 1 day per month, is defined as more than 4 standard drinks for men and more than 3 standard drinks for women during this short period of time. Consequently, alcohol abuse is defined as follows: (a) for men: more than 4 standard drinks on a single occasion or more than 14 standard drinks per week, (b) for women: more than 3 standard drinks on a single occasion or more than 7 standard drinks per week [30].

Defining at-risk levels for alcohol consumption and alcohol abuse is significantly more complicated concerning elderly individuals. There are various important parameters, which should be taken into consideration. Firstly, the burden of used medications, their types, potential interactions with alcohol, polypharmacy, as well as the higher occurrence of physical, psychiatric, and cognitive diseases. Secondly, cultural patterns, sociodemographic factors affecting alcohol intake, such as socioeconomic and marital status, ethnicity and other modifiable risk factors for well-being and healthy aging, such as physical activity, educational level, smoking, and obesity. Finally, there are cognitive, behavioral, and metabolic differences between different age stages above 65 years. As life expectancy has significantly increased globally during the last decades, more caution should be taken regarding those individuals older than 80 years or the oldest old [31].

There are specific recommendations for individuals older than 65 years old. Individual in this age range should consume up to 7 standard drinks per week or less than 3 standard drinks on one single occasion [30]. Regarding those individuals having physical or psychiatric comorbidities, as, for example, depression, or taking certain medications or combining a lot of different pills, it is highly recommended to abstain from drinking alcohol or limit consumption as much as possible. It is also noticed that drinking within recommended levels might not totally disappear the risk for falls, accidents, or deterioration of existing diseases and medical conditions [31].

3.1.5 Pharmacokinetics and Pharmacodynamics

Repeated and long-term consumption is needed for alcohol dependence to be established. In long-term and extensive alcohol use, certain neurochemical procedures occur in specific neuroreceptors and nerve pathways, engaging downregulation of serotonin- and GABA system as well as increased function of glutamate and corticotropin-releasing hormone (CRH) system, leading to addiction. Alcohol can cause certain pharmacological effects which are usually related to concentration levels and can be influenced by genetics, age, and environment. That effect is biphasic; low alcohol intake has a stimulating effect, while high consumption can cause sedation. Alcohol metabolism in older individuals is different than among younger individuals due to changes in liver function and other physiological changes that occur with aging [32]. As people age, alterations occur in their bodies, due to decreased ability to absorb and eliminate alcohol, that can affect how they metabolize and respond to alcohol. Their liver function decreases, and the rate at which alcohol is metabolized slows down. This can lead to increased alcohol levels and higher risk of alcohol-related health complications.

In terms of pharmacokinetics, which is the study of how drugs move through the body, alcohol is absorbed primarily in the small intestine and then enters the bloodstream. The rate of absorption can be affected by several parameters, such as parallel food consumption, amounts of alcohol intake, binge drinking, and the individual's overall health [33]. Once in the bloodstream, alcohol is metabolized mainly in the liver. The physiological mechanisms are related to specific enzymes known as alcohol dehydrogenase and aldehyde dehydrogenase. However, as people age, their liver function may decline and the activity of those enzymes may decrease, which can lead to slower metabolism of alcohol and higher risk of alcohol-related damages [33].

Additionally, alterations in body composition, comprising changes in the proportion of muscle mass and body fat, can also affect alcohol metabolism. The proportion of body fat is higher, while the proportion of lean muscle mass is lower among older individuals. Since alcohol is more soluble in water than fat, this can lead to higher blood alcohol levels in the elderly population. Finally, as people age, their kidneys may become less efficient at eliminating alcohol from the body, which can lead to a longer-lasting and more intense effect of alcohol. Overall, alcohol abuse in the elderly population can have significant health consequences due to changes in pharmacokinetics and the increased risk of alcohol-related harm. It is important for healthcare providers to consider these factors when working with elderly patients with alcohol abuse.

Pharmacodynamics is the study of how drugs, including alcohol, exert their effects on the body. In the case of high alcohol consumption, changes in pharmacodynamics can occur due to a variety of factor. One of the primary factors that can affect alcohol pharmacodynamics in older individuals is a decrease in overall body mass. This can result in a higher blood alcohol concentration (BAC) after consuming the same amount of alcohol as a younger, larger individual. As a result, elderly individuals may experience alcohol-related impairments or aggravation of chronic diseases, such as decreased cardiovascular and liver function, as well as other conditions such as malnutrition, at lower levels of consumption than younger individuals [34]. Changes in brain function can also affect the pharmacodynamics of alcohol in the elderly population. It can lead to increased risk of falls and other accidents. Furthermore, alcohol can interact with certain medications commonly prescribed to elderly individuals, such as benzodiazepines and opioids, which can amplify the effects of alcohol and increase the risk of adverse outcomes. Finally, chronic alcohol overconsumption can lead to significant changes in the brain and other organs, which can further affect pharmacodynamics. For example, chronic alcohol use can lead to cognitive impairment, liver damage, and increased susceptibility to infection. Overall, the pharmacodynamics of high alcohol intake in the elderly population can have significant consequences, including higher risk of falls and other accidents, interactions with medications, and the development of chronic health conditions [35].

3.2 Negative Effect of Alcohol Abuse in Older Individuals

3.2.1 Increased Sensitivity to Alcohol

Elderly individuals may experience an increased sensitivity to alcohol due to age-related changes in their bodies. As people age, their bodies may become less efficient at metabolizing alcohol, which can lead to higher blood alcohol levels and more pronounced effects from drinking. This is because the liver, which is responsible for breaking down alcohol, may not function as well as it did when the person was younger. In addition, elderly individuals may have a decreased ability to tolerate the physical and psychological effects of alcohol due to changes in their brain and nervous system. These changes can make them more susceptible to alcohol-related problems such as falls, confusion, and memory loss. Moreover, elderly individuals are more likely to be taking multiple medications, some of which may interact with alcohol and increase its effects. This can further increase the risk of adverse reactions to alcohol [36].

3.2.2 Dehydration

Alcohol abuse in elderly individuals can lead to dehydration for several reasons. One of the main reasons is that alcohol can have diuretic effect, meaning that it increases urine production and can cause dehydration. This effect is more pronounced in elderly individuals because their bodies may have a decreased ability to conserve water, and their kidneys may not function as efficiently as they did when they were younger. Additionally, elderly individuals may have a decreased sense of thirst, which can make them less likely to drink enough water to stay hydrated. This can be compounded by alcohol use, as it can interfere with the body's normal thirst signals and lead to further dehydration. Dehydration can have serious negative effects on the health of elderly individuals, including confusion, dizziness, and an increased risk of falls [37]. It is important for elderly individuals who abuse alcohol to be aware of the potential for dehydration and to take steps to stay hydrated, such as drinking plenty of water and avoiding alcohol or limiting their alcohol intake. They should also speak with their healthcare provider if they are experiencing symptoms of dehydration or have concerns about their alcohol use.

3.2.3 Increased Health Problems

High alcohol consumption can worsen health problems and burden of comorbidities that elderly people experience. However, there is a high degree of heterogeneity in the literature regarding alcohol research and particularly regarding the association between alcohol consumption and neurocognitive disorders as well as somatic and psychiatric comorbidities [38]. The observed heterogeneity can be explained by some limitations: (a) The assessment method of alcohol consumption has always been self-reported and the majority of studies assessed current drinking, instead of using specific tools and questionnaires controlling for lifetime alcohol consumption [39], (b) there is a wide variety of definition of level, categories, and patterns of alcohol intake due to different size of standard drink and different cultural characteristics across different countries and continents, leading to inadequate standardization of alcohol consumption [40], (c) there is an inadequate control for confounding parameters and interactions between alcohol and clinically relevant factors [41], (d) there are methodological difficulties in separating individuals with former alcohol consumption from lifetime abstainers, which leads to the formation of suboptimal groups of alcohol consumption, (e) finally, the relationship between alcohol and cognitive decline can be negatively influenced by the fact that there is an underrepresentation of individuals with alcohol abuse due to methodological reasons (exclusion criteria) or due to their decreased motivation to participate in research projects. Moreover, those individuals having no medications or severe diseases are more likely to consume higher amounts of alcohol, compared to older individuals with higher burden of drugs and comorbidities [42].

The most basic health conditions are as follows:

Diabetes: While consumption of low to moderate levels of alcohol can be beneficial by increasing insulin sensitivity, alcohol abuse can be one of the most important risk factors for the development of diabetes mellitus [43, 44]. In particular, high alcohol consumption can lead to insulin resistance by negatively affecting the metabolism of glucose. Moreover, it can worsen diabetes-related complications, such as neuropathy and retinopathy. Older individuals with high-alcohol consumption may have suboptimal control over their medications and reduced awareness of the risk of hypoglycemia. Alcohol abuse in older people can increase the risk of developing type 2 diabetes or worsen the symptoms of existing diabetes. Excessive alcohol consumption can affect the body's ability to regulate blood sugar levels, leading to insulin resistance and hyperglycemia. Older adults who abuse alcohol are at higher risk of developing obesity, which can lead to insulin resistance and higher risk of type 2 diabetes [43]. For older adults who have developed diabetes, and also abuse alcohol, it is important to manage both conditions in a coordinated way. This may involve medication management, dietary changes, and alcohol treatment programs tailored to the individual's needs and preferences. Older adults with diabetes who consume alcohol should limit their intake to light to moderate levels. However, some older adults may need to avoid alcohol altogether due to their individual health status or medication use [44].

Hypertension: High alcohol consumption increases the risk for development of hypertension and decreases the effect of antihypertensive treatment. Alcohol abuse in older people can contribute to the development and exacerbation of hypertension. Hypertension is a common condition in older individuals, and excessive alcohol consumption can increase the risk of developing it, as well as worsen its symptoms. Alcohol consumption causes a temporary increase in blood pressure, which can become chronic with excessive drinking. Long-term alcohol abuse can also damage the blood vessels and the heart muscle, leading to a more sustained increase in blood pressure. Moreover, alcohol can negatively influence the effectiveness of blood pressure medications, making it harder to manage hypertension in older adults [43].

Cardiovascular diseases: Alcohol abuse in older people can increase the risk of developing cardiovascular diseases, such as heart disease, stroke, and atrial fibrillation. This is due to the direct effects of alcohol on the cardiovascular system, as well as the indirect effects of alcohol on other risk factors for cardiovascular disease. Alcohol can cause damage to the heart muscle, which can lead to heart failure, and it can increase the levels of triglycerides in the blood, which can contribute to atherosclerosis and increase the risk of heart attack and stroke. Moreover, alcohol abuse can lead to the development of atrial fibrillation, which is a type of irregular heartbeat that increases the risk of stroke and other cardiovascular events. Older adults who abuse alcohol are at higher risk of developing atrial fibrillation than those who drink in moderation or abstain from alcohol [45]. To prevent cardiovascular diseases in older adults who abuse alcohol, healthcare providers should screen for alcohol abuse and provide counseling on the safe limits of alcohol consumption. They should also monitor the cardiovascular health of older adults who abuse alcohol and provide appropriate treatment for hypertension, high cholesterol, and other risk factors. Finally, they should encourage older adults to adopt a healthy lifestyle (physical activity, appropriate diet, and stress-reduction techniques).

Osteoporosis: Alcohol abuse in older people can increase the risk of osteoporosis, by negatively affecting the body's ability to absorb calcium and vitamin D. In addition, alcohol abuse can increase the levels of the hormone cortisol, which can contribute to bone loss. Older adults who abuse alcohol are at higher risk of developing osteoporosis than those who drink in moderation or abstain from alcohol. Moreover, if they have already developed osteoporosis, alcohol abuse can worsen their symptoms and increase the risk of fractures [46].

Gastrointestinal diseases: Alcohol abuse can have a significant impact on gastrointestinal (GI) health in the elderly population. Chronic alcohol use can increase the risk of developing a range of GI diseases, including gastritis, peptic ulcers, and gastrointestinal bleeding. Chronic alcohol use can damage the stomach lining, leading to the development of gastritis. In the elderly population, gastritis can be particularly dangerous because it can increase the risk of bleeding and other complications [47]. Peptic ulcers are sores that can develop in the stomach or duodenum (the first part of the small intestine). Chronic alcohol use can increase the risk of developing peptic ulcers, and it can also exacerbate existing ulcers. Peptic ulcers can cause gastrointestinal symptoms such as nausea, and vomiting, and in severe cases, they can lead to bleeding and perforation of the stomach or duodenum. In severe cases, gastrointestinal bleeding can be life-threatening [48]. Treatment for GI diseases in the elderly population may involve medication management, dietary changes, and, in some cases, endoscopic or surgical interventions. However, the outcomes for elderly patients with these conditions can be poor, and the mortality rate is often high.

Body mass index (BMI) and obesity: There is some evidence to suggest that there may be a relationship between alcohol abuse and body mass index (BMI) in the elderly population. Alcohol is high in calories and can contribute to weight gain, particularly in individuals who consume it regularly and in large amounts. Elderly individuals who abuse alcohol may be at increased risk of obesity or overweight due to the caloric intake from alcohol. Chronic alcohol abuse can lead to nutritional deficiencies, which can also impact BMI. For example, individuals who abuse alcohol may have inadequate intake of protein, vitamins, and minerals, which can contribute to weight loss and malnutrition. Elderly individuals who abuse alcohol may also have underlying health conditions that impact BMI, such as liver disease or diabetes. Physical activity is an important component of maintaining a healthy BMI, but elderly individuals who abuse alcohol may be less likely to engage in regular physical activity due to the impact of alcohol on their physical and mental health. Thus, there may be a relationship between alcohol abuse and BMI in the elderly population [49].

Liver failure: Alcohol overconsumption can have significant consequences for liver health, particularly in the elderly population. Chronic alcohol use can lead to the development of liver disease, which can progress to liver failure. High alcohol consumption can increase the risk for development of cirrhosis and hepatocellular cancer. Inflammatory diseases, such as hepatitis, can worsen even with lower to moderate amounts of alcohol. In the early stages of liver disease, the liver may be able to regenerate and repair itself to some extent. However, as the disease progresses, this ability is diminished, and the liver may become scarred and damaged. This condition is known as cirrhosis and can be a precursor to liver failure [50]. In the elderly population, chronic alcohol use can increase the risk of developing liver disease, and it can also exacerbate existing liver conditions. This is because, as people age, the liver's ability to metabolize alcohol and other substances can decrease, making it more susceptible to damage. Liver failure is a serious condition that can have a range of symptoms, including fatigue, jaundice, abdominal pain, and confusion. In severe cases, liver failure can lead to hepatic encephalopathy, which is a condition characterized by confusion, disorientation, and potentially life-threatening complications [50]. Treatment for liver failure in the elderly population may involve hospitalization, medication management, and, in some cases, a liver transplant. However, the outcomes for elderly patients with liver failure can be poor, and the mortality rate is often high.

Kidney failure: Alcohol overconsumption can have negative consequences for kidney health, particularly in the elderly population. Chronic alcohol use can lead to the development of kidney disease, which can progress to kidney failure. In particular, chronic alcohol use can damage the blood vessels and tissues in the kidneys, leading to reduced kidney function. In the elderly population, chronic alcohol use can increase the risk of developing kidney disease, and it can also exacerbate existing kidney conditions. This is because, as people age, the kidneys' ability to filter blood and eliminate waste can decrease, making them more susceptible to damage. Kidney failure is a serious condition that can have a range of symptoms, including fatigue, swelling, high blood pressure, and changes in urine output. In severe cases, kidney failure can lead to life-threatening complications such as fluid buildup, electrolyte imbalances, and heart failure [51].

Epileptic activity: Alcohol can be a risk factor for the development of seizures, particularly among older individuals with pre-existing intracerebral infarcts, bleeding, or other neurological conditions. In addition, increased epileptic activity can also be related to alcohol withdrawal. Particular caution is needed for individuals, having treatment with antiepileptic medications [52].

For people with epilepsy, alcohol abuse can also worsen their seizures and interfere with the effectiveness of their medication. Elderly individuals with epilepsy should be especially cautious about alcohol use, as alcohol can increase the risk of falls and other accidents, which can be particularly dangerous for older adults. In addition, alcohol can interact with antiepileptic medications, making them less effective and increasing the risk of seizures [53].

Cognitive disorders: Prolonged and extensive alcohol consumption can lead to brain damage, cognitive disorders, and psychological deficits [54]. High alcohol consumption is associated with increased risk for dementia [55]. When it comes to Alzheimer's disease (AD), alcohol is considered to be a contributing factor in around 10% of the most severe cases; however, prevalence varies due to poorly defined diagnostic criteria. The relationship is complex, and some epidemiological studies claim that alcohol in low to moderate amounts can have a protective effect on the development of AD [56]. However, it is unclear whether the findings reflect selection effects in cohort studies or a direct protective effect of alcohol in older people [57]. Nevertheless, identification of specific risk levels for the development of cognitive impairment has been difficult to establish, and the results of ongoing research are still contradictory [57]. This applies in particular to the possible protective effect of light to moderate drinking. According to the literature, the presence of alcohol abuse (AUD) is strongly related to dementia [58]. In addition, a higher prevalence of alcohol-related cognitive impairment and dementia is observed among individuals with early-onset dementia [58]. The fact that light to moderate consumption is associated with a lower risk of dementia has not been able to be definitely confirmed, probably mainly due to methodological reasons [59]. In particular, there is uncertainty as to whether it is truly due to a protective effect or whether it is due to the fact that light to moderate drinking is more common among individuals with higher socioeconomic status and better quality of life [60]. Moreover, it has been shown that a high degree of regional brain atrophy including atrophy in the hippocampus region was observed in individuals with moderate drinking, which indicates that the harmful effect of alcohol exists even at lower levels [61]. Regarding high consumption, there is a consensus in the literature that cognitive impairment and development of dementia occur to a significantly higher degree compared to lower consumption levels [55].

But alcohol has also given its name to a particular form of dementia. The diagnosis of alcohol-related dementia can be set when Alzheimer's disease, vascular dementia, and other dementia types can be ruled out, while individuals with alcohol abuse meets the current criteria for dementia. Typical symptoms of alcohol-related dementia are memory loss, impaired attention, and executive functions (ability to plan and solve problems). Difficulties in orientation are also common, while functions linked to language tend to be relatively intact [62].

Chronic alcohol abuse can also lead to Korsakoff's syndrome, which is related to B1 vitamin deficiency and is characterized by severe memory impairment. Sometimes we talk about Wernicke-Korsakoff syndrome where Wernicke encephalopathy can be a precursor to Korsakoff syndrome. Wernicke encephalopathy is an acute condition caused by deficiency of vitamin B1 (thiamine), a common consequence of alcohol abuse [62]. It is also related to low dietary intake and malnutrition, which is a common problem among older individuals. Confusion, balance difficulties (ataxia), and visual deficits are typical symptoms. Those symptoms are usually transient if the vitamin deficiency is treated in good time. Otherwise, the person may develop Korsakoff's syndrome, a chronic condition that leads to a marked deterioration of short-term memory. The memory impairment in Korsakoff's syndrome appears suddenly, compared to Alzheimer's disease where the memory deficits progress stealthily and gradually increase.

Alcohol-related dementia can occur both with and without Korsakoff's syndrome. In both cases, there is no cure. The positive thing is that the condition does not need to worsen, unlike other dementia types [62]. This assumes that the person immediately stops drinking alcohol. Alcohol-related dementia often has an early onset. It is estimated to be one of the most common among people under the age of

65, but the prevalence remains high among older individuals with continuing alcohol abuse [63].

That type of dementia is underdiagnosed. Since alcohol intake affects the objective character of the procedure of memory investigation, this can only be started after the individual has been alcohol-free for at least 4 months. For many alcohol abusers, it can be perceived as an insurmountable obstacle. Another reason for underdiagnosis is that alcohol-related dementia lacks clear and validated diagnostic criteria, in contrast to, for example, Alzheimer's. Physicians therefore often avoid setting the diagnosis and instead choose the term" unspecified dementia" with the addition that the condition was probably influenced by high alcohol intake [62].

The single most important treatment measure for alcohol-related dementia is for the person to stop drinking alcohol. The deterioration of the cognitive functions can then cease. However, there are no medications that can alleviate the symptoms. The drugs cholinesterase inhibitors and memantine used in Alzheimer's disease have no effect in alcohol-related dementia.

In addition to memory loss and other cognitive deficits, behavioral and psychological symptoms (BPSD) may occur. Those symptoms can be a great nuisance and challenge for healthcare professionals to manage. BPSD should primarily be treated with non-pharmacological measures and appropriate nursing strategies. Medications should be avoided as much as possible.

Psychiatric disorders: Alcohol can worsen depressive symptoms. According to the literature, older individuals quitting dinking and maintaining abstinence experience significant improvement of depressed mood and quality of life. Alcohol can also cause sleep disorders as well as breathing problems while sleeping [64]. Alcohol abuse and depression are common issues among older adults, and there is a complex relationship between the two. While alcohol use can temporarily alleviate symptoms of depression, long-term alcohol abuse can actually worsen depression and lead to other physical and mental health problems.

Older adults who experience symptoms of depression may turn to alcohol as a way to self-medicate and cope with their emotions [65]. However, alcohol can actually worsen symptoms of depression and anxiety over time. Alcohol abuse can alter brain chemistry and lead to changes in mood and behavior. This can contribute to the development or worsening of depression in older adults. Alcohol abuse can also lead to physical health problems, such as liver disease and cardiovascular problems, which can further contribute to feelings of depression and anxiety. Older adults who abuse alcohol may become socially isolated, which can exacerbate feelings of depression and loneliness. It is important for healthcare professionals and addiction specialists to recognize the link between alcohol abuse and depression in older adults and provide integrated treatment that addresses both issues.

3.2.4 Interactions with Medications

Alcohol abuse in older people can have significant interactions with medications. As people age, they may be prescribed multiple medications to manage various health conditions, and the combination of alcohol and these medications can be dangerous [66]. Alcohol can interact with medications in several ways. It can interfere with the metabolism and absorption of medications, leading to increased or decreased effects. It can also increase the risk of side effects, including drowsiness, dizziness, and impaired coordination. In some cases, alcohol can even worsen the underlying medical condition for which the medication is being taken [64]. The prevalence of combination of high alcohol consumption with medications has increased rapidly during the last decades, related to higher rate of alcohol intake among elderly as well as prevalence of polypharmacy and chronic diseases which increases with aging [66]. All observed negative effects are associated with age-related body alterations causing dysfunction in metabolism and distribution of those medications as well as higher rate of brain vulnerability. Moreover, older individuals have higher disease burden, which can be negatively affected of alcohol overconsumption, and deteriorating homeostasis function. Interaction effects can appear with light to moderate alcohol consumption, but become greater with alcohol abuse. There is a wide variety of mechanisms engaging metabolic alterations leading to aggravation of potential side effects and reduction of the therapeutical potential which certain medications have as well as increased levels of alcohol in the bloodstream [64].

Consumed alcohol is initially metabolized in the stomach by the function of alcohol dehydrogenase. Levels of alcohol dehydrogenase are decreasing with age [67]. The rest of the alcohol is being absorbed from the stomach and the small intestine and transported to liver to be partially metabolized. Remaining alcohol enters the bloodstream and is being transported to other organs of the body. All those quantities of alcohol will return to the liver to be metabolized at a later stage. There are medications negatively affecting the function of alcohol dehydrogenase such as aspirin, cimetidine, and ranitidine and other promoting the quicker transport of alcohol through the stomach such as metoclopramide and thus contributing to higher alcohol levels in the bloodstream [64].

Older individuals have lower content of body water and higher content of fat in comparison with younger adults and consequently alcohol is being distributed in a more limited area [14]. Thus, the same amounts of alcohol being transferred to the blood stream after the first phase of metabolism in the liver can correspond to higher alcohol levels in blood among elderly compared with younger individuals. Taking into consideration the fact that specific medications, such as benzodiazepines, that are soluble in fat, have higher distribution areas among older individuals, and consequently more extended half-lives, a combined dynamic effect between alcohol and those medications can be created, increasing the sedative effect and other secondary negative consequences among older individuals [64].

Alcohol is metabolized mainly in the liver. There is a wide variety of enzymes engaged in that procedure [50]. The most important enzymes are those belonging to the cytochrome P450 system. While normal activity of that system is needed for alcohol metabolism of light to moderate intake, significantly higher activity rate is demonstrated related to heavy and extensive chronic alcohol consumption [68]. In addition, those enzymes can not only metabolize alcohol, but also even certain medications, such as benzodiazepines, phenytoin, and warfarin. Therefore, in case of chronic high alcohol consumption, high activity of P450 system can lead to quicker breakdown of those medications and consequently to lower blood concentration. On the contrary, in case of episodic (short-term) heavy drinking, the function of P450 system is mainly focused on alcohol metabolism, leading indirectly to higher concentrations of those medications, if taken parallelly with alcohol, in the blood [64].

As a result of the above-mentioned mechanisms, there is a wide variety of interactions between alcohol and certain medications, depending on body alterations related to aging, the amounts of alcohol consumption, the parallel usage of certain categories of medications, and finally the presence of relevant chronic diseases and medical conditions [50]. Usage of H2 blockers among elderly with high alcohol intake can lead to increased levels of alcohol in the bloodstream. Moreover, while high alcohol consumption, during a long period of time, leads to higher rate of metabolism of both alcohol and medications in the liver by the increased activity of P450 system, and consequently to lower concentration of those drugs in the blood, high alcohol consumption during shorter periods of time leads to the opposite result, namely the inhibition of drug metabolism in favor for the quicker metabolism of alcohol, leading to higher concentration of those drugs in the blood. Metabolism of drugs with anxiolytic and sedative effect, such as benzodiazepines, and warfarin can be affected by the above-mentioned duration of high alcohol intake. Thus, combination of alcohol with sedatives and sleeping pills can increase the risk of drowsiness, dizziness, and impaired coordination, which can lead to falls and accidents [64].

Furthermore, high alcohol intake can aggravate the treatment effect or create side effects of certain medications. There is higher risk for bleeding associated with the usage of aspirin or NSAIDs and greater sedative effect associated with the usage of anxiolytic medications, antidepressants (alcohol can negatively influence the effectiveness of antidepressant medications and increase the risk of depression and suicidal thoughts), and antihistamines. In addition, it can reduce the therapeutical potential which certain medications have against diseases such as high blood pressure and sleeping- and mood disorders. Alcohol can interact with analgesics such as opioids, increasing the risk of respiratory depression, overdose, and other adverse effects, as well as with anticoagulants such as warfarin, increasing the risk of bleeding. Finally, alcohol can interact with diabetes medications, causing hypoglycemia, which can be dangerous in the elderly population [64].

3.3 Evaluation and Management

3.3.1 Diagnostic Tools

Alcohol use disorder (AUD) is significantly underdiagnosed, neglected, and underreported among older individuals. Health practitioners are usually regarding alcohol as a problem mostly related to younger and middle-aged individuals and they are not sufficiently aware about its consequences, when treating and discussing with older individuals. Moreover, physicians tend to be skeptical, unwilling, or ashamed to screen older individuals for alcohol, while elderly use not to reveal their real alcohol consumption in order to avoid stigma and social consequences. Furthermore, symptoms and conditions related to alcohol are usually being attributed to other alternative conditions or to the effect of age. In addition, polypharmacy and side effects of medications absorb the attention and awareness of physicians during controls in the primary care. Finally, an underestimated factor is the attitude that elderly deserve to have a more tolerant treatment regarding lifestyle choices with respect to their lower life expectancy and their ethical right to determine the content of the quality of their remaining life. Consequently, elderly represent a heterogeneous group, which is difficult to undergo adequate screening and follow-up [69].

Moreover, after the Covid-19 pandemic, the rate of depression and loneliness has significantly increased posing more risks for alcohol and generally substance abuse among older individuals and greater challenges for health care. Healthcare professionals, family members, and caregivers should raise awareness about the harmful effects of excessive alcohol consumption on the physical and mental health of older people, as well as on their social and economic well-being. They should also provide information on safe drinking guidelines and the importance of moderation. There are specific signs, symptoms, and events, which can increase suspicion about eventual alcohol use disorder among elderly [70]. Frequent visits at the emergency room, isolated elevated values in specific blood tests such as mean corpuscular volume (MCV) or transaminases, delirium episodes without other detectable cause, cognitive deficits engaging memory and executive functions without typical dementia-related progress, falls or brain injuries, difficulties in controlling chronic diseases such as hypertension and diabetes despite proper treatment strategies, neglecting follow-up controls and visits within health care can indicate eventual alcohol-related issues and should always lead to relevant screening. It is, thus, important that older individuals are screened annually for alcohol use as part of their general medical controls. In case of high alcohol intake, controls should be more frequently planned. If the screening procedure is difficult to be performed and not adequately reliable answers are received, contact with relatives for further information should be considered [69].

There are several biomarkers that can be used to assess alcohol use and its impact on the body in this population [71]. Gamma-glutamyl transferase (GGT) is an enzyme that is found in high levels in the liver and is involved in the metabolism of alcohol. Elevated levels of GGT in the blood can indicate liver damage, and they are a reliable marker of chronic alcohol overconsumption in the elderly population. Mean corpuscular volume (MCV) is a measure of the size of red blood cells, and it can be elevated in individuals who consume excessive amounts of alcohol. In the elderly population, elevated MCV levels can indicate alcohol abuse and its impact on red blood cell production. Carbohydrate-deficient transferrin (CDT) is a type of transferrin (a protein involved in transporting iron in the blood) that is modified in individuals who consume excessive amounts of alcohol. CDT is a specific biomarker for chronic alcohol use, and it can be used to monitor alcohol consumption in the elderly population. Ethyl glucuronide (EtG) is a metabolite of alcohol that can be detected in urine, hair, or blood samples for up to several days after alcohol consumption. EtG testing can be used to assess recent alcohol use in the elderly population. Aspartate aminotransferase (AST) and alanine aminotransferase (ALT) are enzymes that are found in high levels in the liver, and they can indicate liver damage or disease. Elevated levels of these enzymes in the blood can be a sign of chronic alcohol use and its impact on the liver in the elderly population. Imaging tests (magnetic resonance imaging (MRI), computed tomography (CT) scans, and ultrasound) can be used to assess the impact of alcohol abuse on the liver, the brain, and other organs. These tests can detect liver damage, fatty liver disease, increased brain atrophy or vascular brain damages, and other conditions related to alcohol abuse [71].

There are specific screening instruments for the evaluation of AUD in older adults [72]. CAGE (Cut down, Annoyed, Guilty, Eye opener) questionnaire is a quick and easy to perform tool which consists of four parts and assess lifetime alcohol consumption. The CAGE questionnaire is a brief screening tool that can be used to assess alcohol abuse. The acronym stands for the four questions: Have you ever felt the need to Cut down on your drinking? Have you ever felt Annoyed by criticism of your drinking? Have you ever felt Guilty about your drinking? Have you ever had a drink first thing in the morning (Eye opener) to steady your nerves or get rid of a hangover? A positive response to two or more of these questions indicates a higher likelihood of alcohol abuse. It ca be administered in 2 min, The disadvantages are firstly the fact that binge drinking, a continuously increased problem among elderly, is not part of the assessment and secondly the fact that the test was initially designed for younger individuals and it has not been adequately validated for elderly [73].

The Alcohol Use Disorders Identification Test (AUDIT) is another screening tool for alcohol overconsumption, having adequate reliability and age-adjusted cutoffs for elderly. The AUDIT is a more detailed screening tool that can be used to assess alcohol use and related problems. It consists of 10 questions that cover various aspects of alcohol consumption, including the frequency and quantity of alcohol use, dependence, and related problems. A score of 8 or higher on the AUDIT indicates a higher likelihood of alcohol abuse. It can assess the quantity and frequency of alcohol consumption as well as all alcohol-related signs, symptoms, and conditions that may arise. However, relatively unimpaired cognitive functions, particularly memory, are needed [74].

The Senior Alcohol Misuse Indicator (SAMI) questionnaire consists of five parts with questions focused on alcohol consumption and related symptoms. It is appropriate for geriatric populations, and it can decrease stress, embarrassment, and frustration levels when performed as it is not confrontational [72].

The Short Michigan Alcoholism Screening Test- Geriatric version (SMAST-G) is specially adjusted for the assessment of alcohol disorders in geriatric populations. Apart from information related to alcohol consumption, it assesses potential reasons to AUD as well as symptoms that can be caused. However, preserved cognitive functions of insight and judgment as well as high awareness grade about alcohol problems are needed [75].

Finally, there is need of complementary clinical assessment if the above-mentioned screening tools indicate possible alcohol overconsumption. This assessment includes anamnesis about the specific consumption and relevant symptoms particularly regarding cognitive and psychiatric disorders, information about socio-economic and marital status, heredity, blood tests controlling liver and kidney function, comorbidities, and medications [72].

3.3.2 Treatment

Preventing alcohol abuse in older people requires a multifaceted approach that involves brief interventions, cognitive-behavioral therapy, and programs of social and family support. For older adults who are at risk of developing alcohol abuse, brief interventions can be effective in reducing their drinking levels and preventing the onset of more severe problems. These interventions may include motivational interviewing, counseling, and behavioral therapies tailored to the specific needs and preferences of the individual. Behavioral therapies, such as cognitive-behavioral therapy (CBT) and contingency management, can help individuals identify and change problematic behaviors and thought patterns related to alcohol use [76].

Moreover, older adults may benefit from peer support programs that provide socialization, encouragement, and guidance in reducing their alcohol intake. These programs may be delivered through support groups, community-based organizations, or online platforms. For example, support groups, such as Alcoholics Anonymous (AA), can provide emotional support and encouragement from peers who have also experienced alcohol addiction [77]. In addition, they can benefit from support from family members, friends, or other members of the community. This support can include assistance with transportation, meal preparation, and other daily activities [76]. Finally, follow-up care is essential for patients who have received interventions for alcohol abuse. Healthcare providers should monitor patient's consumption and provide ongoing support and treatment as needed. Lifestyle changes, such as regular exercise, healthy eating habits, and stress management techniques, can improve overall health and reduce the risk of relapse. In conclusion, addressing alcohol abuse in the elderly population requires a multifaceted approach, where planned interventions should be tailored to the individual's unique needs and circumstances [72].

If AUD is not advanced, discussions and educational procedures about the harmful effect of alcohol can be beneficial. Older individuals can acquire information about risks related to alcohol such as falls and traumatic brain injuries, and the negative effect to the function of the brain, liver, and kidney. If screening shows higher grade of AUD, medication-assisted treatment can be effective in managing withdrawal symptoms and reducing the risk of relapse [72]. Treatment should be individually determined and planned taking into consideration the specific amounts of alcohol consumption as well as the age and other social and clinical characteristics of the older individuals [78]. The decision of the appropriate setting (primary care or specialized addiction center) and its form (inpatient or outpatient) should be made after discussion and agreement with each individual separately, taking into consideration the cognitive status, the functional ability, and the burden of comorbidities as well as the use of medications [79]. In case of significant cognitive decline, the role of relatives is important. In case of presence of psychiatric disorders, effective treatment of the psychiatric component, for example depression, should be prioritized to improve the therapeutic potential of detoxification and maintenance of withdrawal [72].

There are certain medications that can be used for the treatment of the AUD in older adults. However, certain caution is needed regarding eventual interactions with other pre-existing medications. Naltrexone, which is an opiate receptor blocker, can effectively decrease grade of alcohol consumption. It can be used of older individuals; however, it is not suitable for those individuals using opioids for chronic pain [80]. Disulfiram causes a direct negative response to alcohol intake, including symptoms such as tachycardia and sudden alterations of blood pressure levels, by inhibiting certain enzymes, such as aldehyde dehydrogenase. It is regarded as less suitable for older populations as it can induce higher risks with respect to comorbidity burden and the need of frequent monitoring [81]. Acamprosate can contribute to the maintenance of abstinence by decreasing the enjoyable feelings related to high alcohol consumption. It causes no harmful effects to the liver function, but there is no adequate evidence in the literature regarding usage of older individuals and particularly of those who have impaired kidney function [82]. Effect of pharmacological treatment should be evaluated with blood tests, particularly those controlling liver and kidney function and parameters in blood status that can reflect current alcohol consumption, as well as cognitive and psychological tests.

Older adults with alcohol dependence may have other health conditions that require treatment, such as depression or anxiety. Integrated treatment that addresses both alcohol dependence and other health conditions can help improve outcomes and reduce the risk of future problems. Treatment for alcohol use in older people often involves a combination of approaches that address both physical and psychological aspects of alcohol dependence. The goal of treatment is to help individuals reduce or stop drinking, improve their overall health and well-being, and prevent future alcohol-related problems [72].

3.4 Ethical Considerations

Alcohol abuse can significantly impact the quality of life of older people, both in terms of their physical and mental health. Chronic alcohol abuse can contribute to a wide range of physical, psychiatric, and cognitive conditions, which can all have a negative impact on the person's quality of life. In addition, alcohol overconsumption can exacerbate age-related health problems and increase the risk of falls and other accidents, which can further impact the quality of life.

Managing alcohol abuse in the elderly population requires an ethical approach that takes into account the unique needs and values of each individual. Elderly patients who abuse alcohol should be treated with respect for their autonomy and the right to make decisions about their own care. Healthcare providers should work with patients to develop care plans that align with their goals and values and respect their choices about their own health. Healthcare providers should ensure that elderly patients who abuse alcohol are fully informed about the risks and benefits of treatment options and have given informed consent before any interventions are undertaken. Healthcare providers should ensure that their interventions are just and equitable, and that elderly patients who abuse alcohol are not subjected to discrimination or stigma. Thus, managing alcohol abuse in the elderly population requires an ethical approach that takes into account the unique needs and values of each individual. Healthcare providers should work with patients to develop care plans that respect their autonomy, provide informed consent, minimize harm, promote well-being, and ensure justice and equity.

Alcohol use at the end of life for older individuals should be carefully considered and managed. In some cases, alcohol may be used to manage symptoms such as pain, anxiety, and depression. An older individual may choose to continue drinking alcohol despite their declining health. In these situations, healthcare providers may work with the individual and their loved ones to manage the risks associated with alcohol use, such as falls, confusion, and interactions with medications. However, it is important to note that excessive alcohol use can make end-of-life care more difficult and may interfere with the individual's ability to receive the care and support they need. It can also increase the risk of adverse events and complications, which can be particularly concerning for older individuals who may already be frail or have multiple chronic conditions.

Alcohol abuse is a significant health concern among the elderly population, and it can be particularly challenging for healthcare providers to manage in palliative care, where the focus is on improving quality of life and managing symptoms [83]. Healthcare providers should work with patients and their families to develop care plans that align with their goals and values. Managing alcohol abuse in palliative care often requires a multidisciplinary approach, involving physicians, nurses, social workers, and other healthcare professionals. Alcohol withdrawal symptoms can be challenging to manage. Healthcare providers should have a plan in place for managing symptoms such as tremors, seizures, and delirium. Family members can play a critical role in supporting elderly patients in the last phase of their life. Healthcare providers should work with families to provide education and support to help them manage the patient's symptoms. In conclusion, a comprehensive, multidisciplinary approach that focuses on improving quality of life and managing symptoms is required.

3.5 Future Perspectives

Alcohol abuse in older people is a growing concern due to the aging population and the potential negative health consequences. It is important to understand the unique perspectives of older adults with regard to alcohol abuse to effectively prevent and address this issue.

One factor to consider is the social and cultural attitudes toward alcohol consumption among older adults. In some cultures, drinking alcohol is a social norm and is viewed as a way to relax and socialize. In addition, older adults may have more leisure time and fewer responsibilities, which may contribute to increased alcohol consumption [14]. Addressing these attitudes and promoting healthy leisure activities can help prevent alcohol abuse in older adults.

Another promising area of research is the development of new interventions to prevent and manage alcohol abuse in the elderly population. This includes strategies such as alcohol screening and brief interventions, which have been shown to be effective in limiting alcohol use and related health problems in older adults [76]. Other interventions under investigation include medication-assisted therapies, behavioral therapies, and online self-help programs.

Another area of research is focused on developing better biomarkers and diagnostic tools for alcohol abuse in the elderly population. These tools can help healthcare providers identify individuals who are at risk of alcohol-related health problems and provide appropriate interventions to prevent or manage these condition. In addition, there is a growing recognition of the importance of addressing social and environmental factors that contribute to alcohol abuse in the elderly population. This includes addressing social isolation, access to healthcare services, and other factors that can increase the risk of alcohol abuse and related health problems in this population [69].

An additional factor to consider is the potential for alcohol abuse to be a symptom of underlying mental health issues such as depression, anxiety, or loneliness. Older adults may experience social isolation and loneliness, which can lead to depression and anxiety, and may turn to alcohol as a treatment alternative. Addressing these underlying mental health issues and providing social support can help prevent alcohol abuse in older adults [65].

Moreover, healthcare providers need to be aware of the unique health concerns and medication interactions that may occur in older adults who abuse alcohol. Older adults may be taking multiple medications, and alcohol can reduce the effectiveness of these medications or exacerbate their side effects [66]. Healthcare providers need to be aware of these risks and provide appropriate counseling and treatment to prevent alcohol abuse and manage any related health concerns.

Finally, there is a need to improve awareness and education about alcohol abuse in the elderly population among healthcare providers, caregivers, and the general public. This includes promoting safe drinking practices and increasing awareness of the risks and consequences of alcohol abuse in older individuals.

In conclusion, future perspectives on alcohol abuse in the elderly population are focused on improving prevention, diagnosis, and treatment of alcohol-related health problems, as well as addressing social and environmental factors that contribute to alcohol abuse in this population. By taking a comprehensive and multidisciplinary approach to this issue, we can improve the health and quality of life of older individuals and reduce the burden of alcohol-related health problems in this population.

References

1. Rigler SK. Alcoholism in the elderly. Am Fam Physician. 2000;61(6):1710–6. 1883–4, 1887–8 passim.
2. Kelly S, Olanrewaju O, Cowan A, Brayne C, Lafortune L. Alcohol and older people: a systematic review of barriers, facilitators and context of drinking in older people and implications for intervention design. PLoS One. 2018;13(1):e0191189.
3. Substance Abuse and Mental Health Services Administration. 2019. https://www.samhsa.gov/data/sites/default/files/reports/rpt29394/NSDUHDetailedTabs2019/NSDUHDetTabsSect2pe2019.htm#tab2-7b. Accessed 23 Mar 2023.
4. Latanioti M, Schuster JP, Rosselet Amoussou J, Strippoli MPF, von Gunten A, Ebbing K, et al. Epidemiology of at-risk alcohol use and associated comorbidities of interest among community-dwelling older adults: a protocol for a systematic review. BMJ Open. 2020;10(1):e035481.
5. Pierucci-Lagha A. Alcoholism and aging. 1. Epidemiology, clinical aspects and treatment. Psychol Neuropsychiatr Vieil. 2003 Sep;1(3):197–205.
6. Hu Y, Pikhart H, Malyutina S, Pajak A, Kubinova R, Nikitin Y, et al. Alcohol consumption and physical functioning among middle-aged and older adults in Central and Eastern Europe: results from the HAPIEE study. Age Ageing. 2015;44(1):84–9.
7. Sanna MB, Tuqan AT, Goldsmith JS, Law MS, Ramirez KD, Liao DH, et al. Characteristics of older at-risk drinkers who drive after drinking and those who do not drive after drinking. Traffic Inj Prev. 2015;16(2):104–8.
8. Bosque-Prous M, Brugal MT, Lima KC, Villalbí JR, Bartroli M, Espelt A. Hazardous drinking in people aged 50 years or older: a cross-sectional picture of Europe, 2011-2013. Int J Geriatr Psychiatry. 2017;32(8):817–28.
9. Anderson P, Scafato E, Galluzzo L, VINTAGE project Working Group. Alcohol and older people from a public health perspective. Ann Ist Super Sanita. 2012;48(3):232–47.
10. Breslow RA, Castle IJP, Chen CM, Graubard BI. Trends in alcohol consumption among older Americans: National Health Interview Surveys, 1997 to 2014. Alcohol Clin Exp Res. 2017;41(5):976–86.
11. Butt PR, White-Campbell M, Canham S, Johnston AD, Indome EO, Purcell B, et al. Canadian guidelines on alcohol use disorder among older adults. Can Geriatr J. 2020;23(1):143–8.
12. Belay GM, Lam KKW, Liu Q, Wu CST, Mak YW, Ho KY. Magnitude and determinants of alcohol use disorder among adult population in East Asian countries: a systematic review and meta-analysis. Front Public Health. 2023;11:1144012.
13. Trangenstein PJ, Morojele NK, Lombard C, Jernigan DH, Parry CDH. Heavy drinking and contextual risk factors among adults in South Africa: findings from the International Alcohol Control study. Subst Abuse Treat Prev Policy. 2018;13(1):43.
14. Sorocco KH, Ferrell SW. Alcohol use among older adults. J Gen Psychol. 2006;133(4):453–67.
15. Nuevo R, Chatterji S, Verdes E, Naidoo N, Ayuso-Mateos JL, Miret M. Prevalence of alcohol consumption and pattern of use among the elderly in the WHO European Region. Eur Addict Res. 2015;21(2):88–96.
16. Collins SE. Associations between socioeconomic factors and alcohol outcomes. Alcohol Res. 2016;38(1):83–94.
17. Shankar A, McMunn A, Steptoe A. Health-related behaviors in older adults relationships with socioeconomic status. Am J Prev Med. 2010;38(1):39–46.
18. Assari S, Lankarani MM. Education and alcohol consumption among older Americans; black–white differences. Front Public Health [Internet]. 2016;4. Available from: https://www.frontiersin.org/articles/10.3389/fpubh.2016.00067.
19. OECD. Tackling harmful alcohol use economics and public health policy: economics and public health policy. Berlin: OECD Publishing; 2015. p. 236.
20. Goldman D, Oroszi G, Ducci F. The genetics of addictions: uncovering the genes. Nat Rev Genet. 2005;6(7):521–32.

21. Merikangas KR, McClair VL. Epidemiology of substance use disorders. Hum Genet. 2012;131(6):779–89.
22. Avenevoli S, Conway KP, Merikangas KR. Chapter 9—Familial risk factors for substance use disorders. In: Hudson JL, Rapee RM, editors. Psychopathology and the family. Oxford: Elsevier; 2005. p. 167–92.
23. Seripa D, Panza F, Daragjati J, Paroni G, Pilotto A. Measuring pharmacogenetics in special groups: geriatrics. Expert Opin Drug Metab Toxicol. 2015;11(7):1073–88.
24. Nolen-Hoeksema S, Hilt L. Possible contributors to the gender differences in alcohol use and problems. J Gen Psychol. 2006;133(4):357–74.
25. Fama R, Le Berre AP, Sullivan EV. Alcohol's unique effects on cognition in women: a 2020 (re)view to envision future research and treatment. Alcohol Res. 2020;40(2):03.
26. Rossow I, Træen B. Alcohol use among older adults: a comparative study across four European countries. Nordic Stud Alcohol Drugs. 2020;37(6):526–43.
27. Stelander LT, Høye A, Bramness JG, Wynn R, Grønli OK. Sex differences in at-risk drinking and associated factors–a cross-sectional study of 8,616 community-dwelling adults 60 years and older: the Tromsø study, 2015-16. BMC Geriatr. 2022;22(1):170.
28. Grace S, Rossetti MG, Allen N, Batalla A, Bellani M, Brambilla P, et al. Sex differences in the neuroanatomy of alcohol dependence: hippocampus and amygdala subregions in a sample of 966 people from the ENIGMA Addiction Working Group. Transl Psychiatry. 2021;11(1):156.
29. Babor TF, Higgins-Biddle JC, Saunders JB, Monteiro MG. AUDIT The Alcohol Use Disorders Identification Test. 2nd ed. WHO. 2001. https://www.who.int/publications/i/item/WHO-MSD-MSB-01.6a. Accessed 29 Mar 2023.
30. "Dietary Guidelines for Americans 2020-2025," U.S. Department of Health and Human Services and U.S. Department of Agriculture, NIAAA The Substance Abuse and Mental Health Services Administration (SAMHSA). 2020. https://www.dietaryguidelines.gov/sites/default/files/2020-12/Dietary_Guidelines_for_Americans_2020-2025.pdf. Accessed 21 Feb 2023.
31. Callinan S, Livingston M, Dietze P, Gmel G, Room R. Age-based differences in quantity and frequency of consumption when screening for harmful alcohol use. Addiction. 2022;117(9):2431–7.
32. Franck J, Nylander I. Beroendemedicin. 3rd ed. Lund: Studentlitteratur AB; 2022.
33. Lal R, Pattanayak RD. Alcohol use among the elderly: issues and considerations. J Geriatr Ment Health. 2017;4(1):4.
34. Kuerbis A, Sacco P, Blazer DG, Moore AA. Substance abuse among older adults. Clin Geriatr Med. 2014;30(3):629–54.
35. Barry KL, Blow FC. Drinking over the lifespan: focus on older adults. Alcohol Res. 2016;38(1):115–20.
36. Wadd S, Papadopoulos C. Drinking behaviour and alcohol-related harm amongst older adults: analysis of existing UK datasets. BMC Res Notes. 2014;7:741.
37. Polhuis KCMM, Wijnen AHC, Sierksma A, Calame W, Tieland M. The diuretic action of weak and strong alcoholic beverages in elderly men: a randomized diet-controlled crossover trial. Nutrients [Internet]. 2017;9(7) https://doi.org/10.3390/nu9070660.
38. Rehm J, Hasan OSM, Black SE, Shield KD, Schwarzinger M. Alcohol use and dementia: a systematic scoping review. Alzheimer's Res Ther. 2019;11(1):1.
39. Xu W, Wang H, Wan Y, Tan C, Li J, Tan L, et al. Alcohol consumption and dementia risk: a dose-response meta-analysis of prospective studies. Eur J Epidemiol. 2017;32:31–42.
40. Ilomaki J, Jokanovic N, Tan ECK, Lonnroos E. Alcohol consumption, dementia and cognitive decline: an overview of systematic reviews. Curr Clin Pharmacol. 2015;10(3):204–12.
41. Marco LYD, Di Marco LY, Marzo A, Muñoz-Ruiz M, Arfan Ikram M, Kivipelto M, et al. Modifiable lifestyle factors in dementia: a systematic review of longitudinal observational cohort studies [Internet]. J Alzheimer's Dis. 2014;42:119–35. https://doi.org/10.3233/jad-132225.
42. Livingston G, Sommerlad A, Orgeta V, Costafreda SG, Huntley J, Ames D, et al. Dementia prevention, intervention, and care. Lancet. 2017;390:2673–734.

43. Heuberger RA. Alcohol and the older adult: a comprehensive review. J Nutr Elder. 2009;28(3):203–35.
44. Carlsson S, Hammar N, Grill V. Alcohol consumption and type 2 diabetes: a meta analyses of epidemiological studies indicates a U shaped relationship. Diabetologia. 2005;48:1051–4.
45. Fernández-Solà J. Cardiovascular risks and benefits of moderate and heavy alcohol consumption. Nat Rev Cardiol. 2015;12(10):576–87.
46. Cheraghi Z, Doosti-Irani A, Almasi-Hashiani A, Baigi V, Mansournia N, Etminan M, et al. The effect of alcohol on osteoporosis: a systematic review and meta-analysis. Drug Alcohol Depend. 2019;197:197–202.
47. Bishehsari F, Magno E, Swanson G, Desai V, Voigt RM, Forsyth CB, et al. Alcohol and gut-derived inflammation. Alcohol Res. 2017;38(2):163–71.
48. Strate LL, Singh P, Boylan MR, Piawah S, Cao Y, Chan AT. A prospective study of alcohol consumption and smoking and the risk of major gastrointestinal bleeding in men. PLoS One. 2016;11(11):e0165278.
49. Traversy G, Chaput JP. Alcohol consumption and obesity: an update. Curr Obes Rep. 2015;4(1):122–30.
50. Meier P, Seitz HK. Age, alcohol metabolism and liver disease. Curr Opin Clin Nutr Metab Care. 2008;11(1):21–6.
51. Kazancioğlu R. Risk factors for chronic kidney disease: an update. Kidney Int Suppl. 2013;3(4):368–71.
52. Qi J, Liu X, Xu N, Wang Q. The clinical characteristics of new-onset epilepsy in the elderly and risk factors for treatment outcomes of antiseizure medications. Front Neurol. 2022;13:819889.
53. Liu S, Yu W, Lü Y. The causes of new-onset epilepsy and seizures in the elderly. Neuropsychiatr Dis Treat. 2016;12:1425–34.
54. Harper C. The neurotoxicity of alcohol. Hum Exp Toxicol. 2007;26(3):PP251–7.
55. Langballe EM, Ask H, Holmen J, Stordal E, Saltvedt I, Selbaek G, Fikseaunet A, Bergh S, Nafstad P, Tambs K. Alcohol consumption and risk of dementia up to 27 years later in a large, population-based sample. The HUNT study, Norway. Eur J Epidemiol. 2015;30:1049–56.
56. Kivipelto M, Solomon A. Alzheimer's disease—the ways of prevention. J Nutr Health Aging. 2008;12(Supplement 1):S89–94.
57. Anstey KJ, Mack HA, Cherbuin N. Alcohol consumption as a risk factor for dementia and cognitive decline: meta-analysis of prospective studies. Am J Geriatr Psychiatry. 2009;17(7):542–55.
58. Schwarzinger M, Pollock BG, OSM H, Dufouil C, Rehm J, QalyDays Study Group. Contribution of alcohol use disorders to the burden of dementia in France 2008-13: a nationwide retrospective cohort study. Lancet Public Health. 2018;3:e124–e32.
59. Verbaten MN. Chronic effects of low to moderate alcohol consumption on structural and functional properties of the brain: beneficial or not? Human Psychopharmacol. 2009;24:199–20.
60. Hersi M, Irvine B, Gupta P, Gomes J, Birkett N, Krewski D. Risk factors associated with the onset and progression of Alzheimer's disease: a systematic review of the evidence. Neurotoxicology. 2017;61:143–87.
61. Topiwala A, Allan CL, Valkanova V, Zsoldos E, Filippini N, Sexton C, et al. Moderate alcohol consumption as risk factor for adverse brain outcomes and cognitive decline: longitudinal cohort study. BMJ. 2017;357:j2353.
62. Ridley N, Droper B, Withall A. Alcohol-related dementia: an update of the evidence. Alzheimer's Res Ther. 2013;5:3.
63. Nordstrom P, Nordstrom A, Eriksson M, Wahlund LO, Gustafson Y. Risk factors in late adolescence for young-onset dementia in men: a nationwide cohort study. JAMA Intern Med. 2013;173:1612–8.
64. Moore AA, Whiteman EJ, Ward KT. Risks of combined alcohol/medication use in older adults. Am J Geriatr Pharmacother. 2007;5(1):64–74.
65. Choi NG, Dinitto DM. Heavy/binge drinking and depressive symptoms in older adults: gender differences. Int J Geriatr Psychiatry. 2011;26(8):860–8.

66. Breslow RA, Faden VB, Smothers B. Alcohol consumption by elderly Americans. J Stud Alcohol. 2003;64(6):884–92.
67. Shimamoto C, Hirata I, Hiraike Y, Takeuchi N, Nomura T, Katsu KI. Evaluation of gastric motor activity in the elderly by electrogastrography and the 13C-acetate breath test. Gerontology. 2002;48(6):381–6.
68. Vestal RE, McGuire EA, Tobin JD, Andres R, Norris AH, Mezey E. Aging and ethanol metabolism. Clin Pharmacol Ther. 1977;21(3):343–54.
69. Taylor MH, Grossberg GT. The growing problem of illicit substance abuse in the elderly: a review. Prim Care Companion CNS Disord [Internet]. 2012;14(4):PCC.11r01320.
70. Satre DD, Hirschtritt ME, Silverberg MJ, Sterling SA. Addressing problems with alcohol and other substances among older adults during the COVID-19 pandemic. Am J Geriatr Psychiatry. 2020;28(7):780–3.
71. Fakhari S, Waszkiewicz N. Old and new biomarkers of alcohol abuse: narrative review. J Clin Med Res [Internet]. 2023;12(6):2124.
72. Joshi P, Duong KT, Trevisan LA, Wilkins KM. Evaluation and management of alcohol use disorder among older adults. Curr Geriatr Rep. 2021;10(3):82–90.
73. Ewing JA. Detecting alcoholism. The CAGE questionnaire. JAMA. 1984;252(14):1905–7.
74. Aalto M, Alho H, Halme JT, Seppä K. The Alcohol Use Disorders Identification Test (AUDIT) and its derivatives in screening for heavy drinking among the elderly. Int J Geriatr Psychiatry. 2011;26(9):881–5.
75. Blow FC, Gillespie BW, Barry KL, Mudd SA, Hill EM. Brief screening for alcohol problems in elderly populations using the Short Michigan Alcoholism Screening Test-Geriatric Version (SMAST-G). Alcohol Clin Exp Res. 1998;22(3):20–5.
76. Schonfeld L, Hazlett RW, Hedgecock DK, Duchene DM, Burns LV, Gum AM. Screening, brief intervention, and referral to treatment for older adults with substance misuse. Am J Public Health. 2015;105(1):205–11.
77. Nicholson NR. A review of social isolation: an important but underassessed condition in older adults. J Prim Prev. 2012;33(2-3):137–52.
78. Friedrichs A, Spies M, Härter M, Buchholz A. Patient preferences and shared decision making in the treatment of substance use disorders: a systematic review of the literature. PLoS One. 2016;11(1):e0145817.
79. Kuerbis A, Sacco P. A review of existing treatments for substance abuse among the elderly and recommendations for future directions. Subst Abuse. 2013;7:13–37.
80. Sinclair JMA, Chambers SE, Shiles CJ, Baldwin DS. Safety and tolerability of pharmacological treatment of alcohol dependence: comprehensive review of evidence. Drug Saf. 2016;39(7):627–45.
81. Le Roux C, Tang Y, Drexler K. Alcohol and opioid use disorder in older adults: neglected and treatable illnesses. Curr Psychiatry Rep. 2016;18(9):87.
82. Witkiewitz K, Saville K, Hamreus K. Acamprosate for treatment of alcohol dependence: mechanisms, efficacy, and clinical utility. Ther Clin Risk Manag. 2012;8:45–53.
83. MacCormac A. Alcohol dependence in palliative care: a review of the current literature. J Palliat Care. 2017;32(3-4):108–12.

Treatment of Challenging Behavior in Dementia

4

Ruslan Leontjevas, Marion Klaver, Martin Smalbrugge, and Debby L. Gerritsen

4.1 Challenging Behavior

In dementia research and care, the behavior of people with dementia has puzzled researchers and professionals for decades. Behaviors considered "challenging"—also referred to as neuropsychiatric symptoms or behavioral and psychological symptoms of dementia—are heterogeneous and may include agitation, apathy, depression, irritability, vocalizations, disinhibition, and sleep problems [1, 2]. Such behaviors can cause suffering or pose a danger to those with dementia and others in their environment [3, 4]. Typically, challenging behavior is ubiquitous across all

R. Leontjevas
Department of Primary and Community Care, Radboud University Medical Center, Radboud Research Institute for Medical Innovation, Radboud Alzheimer Center, Nijmegen, The Netherlands

Faculty of Psychology, Open University of The Netherlands, Heerlen, The Netherlands
e-mail: Roeslan.leontjevas@ou.nl

M. Klaver
Department of Medicine for Older People, location Vrije Universiteit Amsterdam, Amsterdam University Medical Center, Amsterdam, The Netherlands

Zorggroep Amsterdam Oost, Amsterdam, The Netherlands
e-mail: m.g.klaver@amsterdamumc.nl

M. Smalbrugge
Department of Medicine for Older People, location Vrije Universiteit Amsterdam, Amsterdam University Medical Center, Amsterdam, The Netherlands

Amsterdam Public Health Research Institute, Aging & Later Life, Amsterdam, Netherlands
e-mail: m.smalbrugge@amsterdamumc.nl

D. L. Gerritsen (✉)
Department of Primary and Community Care, Radboud University Medical Center, Radboud Research Institute for Medical Innovation, Radboud Alzheimer Center, Nijmegen, The Netherlands
e-mail: debby.gerritsen@radboudumc.nl

N. Veronese, A. Marseglia (eds.), *Psychogeriatrics*, Practical Issues in Geriatrics,
https://doi.org/10.1007/978-3-031-58488-6_4

types of dementia and at all stages of the disease [5]. More than 50% of people with dementia living at home and over 80% of nursing home residents will develop one or more behavioral alterations. As dementia progresses, challenging behavior often becomes more severe [2, 6–8].

Challenging behavior negatively affects the well-being of people with dementia and is associated with increased mortality [9]. It is reported being more stressful for caregivers than cognitive or functional decline [10]. Family caregivers often experience more distress, desperation, isolation [11], and poorer physical and mental health than their peers [12]. In nursing homes, challenging behavior can cause distress in other residents and care staff [8]. The compromised well-being of people living with dementia and others in their social environment, caused by challenging behavior, has prompted clinicians to urgently seek effective interventions. These interventions should focus not only on people with dementia but also on family members and professional caregivers, as they can both be affected by and play a role in causing and sustaining challenging behavior.

Some types of challenging behavior are strongly associated with specific types of dementia, suggesting a (neuro-)biological origin. For example, depression is more common in vascular dementia, while wandering and socially inappropriate behavior are more frequently seen in frontotemporal dementia [13]. Additionally, certain modifiable and non-modifiable psychological, social, and environmental factors may cause challenging behavior [14]. For instance, an unhealthy diet can result in deficiencies of nutrients needed for a healthy brain. Challenging behavior can also be associated with pain, chronic stress, age-related or acute health conditions, poor education, personality traits, stigma, low socioeconomic status, or limited access to resources [13].

Associations between challenging behavior and modifiable factors can inform hypothesis-driven research on new interventions. Non-modifiable factors (e.g., age or biological sex) can be potential moderators of intervention effects and need to be considered in research and clinical practice.

4.2 Theoretical Approaches

There are various theoretical approaches to challenging behavior. According to learning theory, challenging behavior can increase when it receives attention from the social environment (e.g., paying attention to yelling may cause yelling to increase, while ignoring it may result in its reduction) [15]. Another approach focuses on the neurobiological nature of behavior, regarding challenging behavior as a symptom of brain damage in dementia. A third way to look at challenging behavior is to see it as a means of communication [16] or a signal that has a function: a signal related to unfulfilled needs [17].

Function-focused approaches to challenging behavior include the unmet-needs approach [18], the lowered-threshold theory [19], and Dröes' adaptation-coping model [20, 21]. The unmet-needs approach posits three needs-related causes of challenging behavior: (1) the behavior is an expression of distress caused by unmet needs, (2) the behavior is a way of communicating an unmet need, or (3) the behavior manifests needs being fulfilled in a way that others perceive as challenging [18]. For instance, a hungry person may aggressively take food from another person. The lowered-threshold model proposes that challenging behavior results from exceeding a stress threshold. This threshold is considered to decrease progressively in people with dementia due to their increased vulnerability to stimuli caused by neurological damage [19, 22]. According to Droës' adaptation-coping model [21], challenging behavior is an attempt by people with dementia to cope with their condition and make sense of the world as they experience it.

An eclectic approach combines different theories and models. This approach is widely used in dementia care. It can provide a more comprehensive understanding of the causes of challenging behavior and the working mechanisms of effective interventions than any single theory or model. For example, music therapy generates positive attention from staff members (learning theory), fulfills the need for creative and pleasant activities, and provides an optimal level of stimulation [15]. Several international and national guidelines, such as those from the International Psychogeriatric Association [15], NICE (National Institute for Health and Care Excellence; UK) [23], and the National Health Service in the UK and Verenso in the Netherlands [24, 25] can be considered eclectic. These guidelines do not focus on one specific theory but rather emphasize the importance of a systematical (methodic) approach to treating challenging behavior.

4.3 A Stepwise Cyclic Approach

One way to work systematically is by using the methodical cycle. This cycle commonly consists of four phases: (1) Describing, detecting, and measuring the behavior in its environmental context; (2) establishing priorities and analyzing possible causes and consequences; (3) choosing and conducting treatment based on a clear treatment goal, formulating specific actions to reach the goal, clarifying who will execute which actions, and agreeing on when the treatment should be evaluated; and (4) monitoring and evaluating the treatment results, which may result in either the continuation or adjustment of the treatment. Examples of methodological approaches can be found in programs such as Grip on Challenging Behavior [26]; DICE, Describe, Investigate, Create, and Evaluate [5]; and TIME, Targeted Interdisciplinary Model for Evaluation and Treatment of Neuropsychiatric Symptoms [27].

4.3.1 Phase 1: Describe and Measure

In Phase 1, the use of a validated instrument is recommended. This can harmonize communication between professionals and enable assessment comparison with other patients, with existing literature and norms or across several measurements concerning the individual with dementia. Examples of such instruments are the Neuropsychiatric Inventory Questionnaire (NPI-Q) [28] and BEHAVE-AD [29]. If necessary, an instrument for a specific "behavior" can be used, such as the Apathy Evaluation Scale (AES) [30], the Cornell Scale for Depression in Dementia [31], or the Cohen-Mansfield Agitation Inventory [32]. A scale like NPI-Q is useful not only for evaluating which challenging behavior is present, but also for establishing caregivers burden.

When possible, the validated instruments should combine information from different sources such as observations by others and self-reports from the patient. Caregivers might attenuate problems reported by people with dementia [33]. This means that observers may perceive problems as less severe (e.g., extreme sleeping problems as reported by the patient) or may report more severe problems when the patient reports almost none.

4.3.2 Phase 2: Prioritize and Analyze

Once the challenging behavior has been identified and measured, the results of Phase 1 can help prioritize those problems that are especially burdensome for the individual with dementia or very demanding for others involved in daily care (e.g., professional caregivers and family) or in daily life (e.g., family and other residents in a nursing home). Certain behaviors can be dangerous for the person or others and must be prioritized for treatment.

Establishing priorities involves prioritizing not only specific challenging behaviors but also their causes. According to various guidelines, before planning any treatment, it is essential to address easily modifiable discomforting factors related to the individual with dementia, the caregiver, and the environment [15]. For this, the causes and aspects that maintain or exacerbate challenging behavior need to be explored. First, a review of the medication status is necessary. Starting a new medication or withdrawing from previously used medication may precede the onset of specific behaviors. Furthermore, a physical examination should be conducted to determine whether fever, inflammation, or any abdominal or other types of pain might explain or prolong challenging behavior. Other health-related factors that need to be addressed include incontinence and poor vision or hearing [15, 34].

In addition to factors related to people with dementia, caregiver factors also need to be prioritized. These may include (unrealistic) expectations, caregiving style, and available resources. Environmental factors can encompass over- or under-stimulation, available activities, structure, and safety issues [16].

Some aspects may remain unclear at this phase. As previously mentioned, a theoretical approach can assist in prioritizing which factors to focus on in an intervention.

4.3.3 Phase 3: Intervene

When selecing and implementing treatment strategies in Phase 3, it is recommended to follow a stepwise approach. This approach advices using pharmacological treatment only when non-pharmacological treatments have proven unsuccessful. This recommendation aligns with expert groups and several guidelines, including international good practice guidelines [5, 13, 16, 35, 36]. In practice, a pharmacological approach may be chosen as the first treatment when other interventions are not feasible. For behavior deemed extremely burdensome or even dangerous, a combination of both non-pharmacological and pharmacological treatments could be considered.

A Cochrane meta-analysis on challenging behavior which included results of seven reviews on pharmacological interventions and eight reviews on non-pharmacological interventions concluded that functional analysis-based interventions should be used as first-line treatment [35]. Examples of these interventions include Dementia-Care-Mapping, a method for measuring the experiences of people with dementia to guide ongoing improvements in person-centered care [36]. This person-centered care is considered the gold standard of care. It adopts an eclectic approach, supporting the individual's abilities while recognizing the importance of their personality, preferences, and history [37].

Recent meta-analyses have confirmed the positive effects of person-centered care on challenging behavior [36, 38]. Professionals and caregivers addressing challenging behavior can refer to existing evidence on specific strategies for providing person-centered care. Subsequent paragraphs will delve into the evidence supporting non-pharmacological and pharmacological strategies.

4.3.4 Phase 4: Evaluate

This phase includes a thorough evaluation of the intervention elements and monitoring of the observed effects. Measurements are needed during the treatment, immediately after the treatment, and several months after that to determine whether an achieved change is permanent and/or whether adjustments in the intervention are necessary.

It is important to realize that each intervention can be considered a complex procedure involving different elements. For instance, an activity-based intervention might include a music intervention in a group. The effects can be attributed to listening to sounds, dancing (involving physical movements), social interaction, tactile experiences (e.g., when using an instrument), and distraction. Even pharmacological interventions cannot be regarded as simple interventions, as interaction is always a possibility with the professional who prescribes or provides the medication. Furthermore, it is important to realize that the assessment and diagnostic procedure can stimulate additional actions in people with dementia or other individuals from their social environment [39].

Actions taken by the person with dementia or those significant to them can be executed either intentionally or unintentionally after the diagnostic procedure. For instance, intentional actions might include taking the person with dementia for regular walks in the park. On the other hand, unintentional actions might involve caregivers altering the tone of their voices when approaching a person with challenging behavior. Such actions alongside formal treatment strategies can affect outcomes, so it is prudent to monitor them. However, up to the present, little research has been conducted on these informal activities and their effects. A promising instrument has been developed for assessing residents with depressive symptoms in nursing homes [40]. For other challenging behaviors, observations and in-depth interviews with those involved in the daily care and life of people with dementia can be used. These observations and interviews also play a crucial role in evaluating treatment effects. For the latter, instruments that were described for phase 2 can provide insight into whether the intervention was successful. Nonetheless, these tools should be sensitive to changes in addition to their ability to identify problems, which was the main focus of Phase 2.

4.4 Non-pharmacological Interventions

As previously mentioned, non-pharmacological interventions are recommended as the first-line treatment for challenging behavior. Such interventions can be provided by a professional therapist (e.g., a psychotherapist) using "talk" therapy or by staff members and family members without extensive training. One example of basic non-pharmacological intervention is modifying the physical environment. This can be prescribed by a therapist but implemented by professionals or family members who have not received specific training to handle challenging behavior. Section 4.4 presents empirical evidence on basic non-pharmacological interventions, and on psychotherapeutic approaches supervised or provided by a psychologist or psychotherapist. If a multidisciplinary team is available, a combination of several (evidence-based) interventions can be considered.

4.4.1 Stimulation-Oriented Treatments

Stimulation-oriented therapies can be appealing in practice due to their feasibility in both severe and less severe dementia. This cluster of non-pharmacological interventions does not require active cognitive work from the individual with dementia.

4.4.1.1 Sensory Stimulation

Sensory stimulation represents one type of non-pharmacological interventions. A recent review provided the strongest and most persistent evidence to date that music interventions can be used to reduce challenging behavior [36]. Music intervention is an example of an intervention involving sensory stimulation. Research on other forms of sensory stimulation therapies, such as aromatherapy, *snoezelen*, and light interventions, indicated that these may also be beneficial for mitigating challenging behavior [41, 42]. However, aromatherapy and touch therapy displayed inconclusive, albeit non-harmful results, while light therapy was potentially effective but should be used with caution as it might increase agitation [43].

4.4.1.2 Physical Activity and Exercise [44]

A literature review [41] that integrated both qualitative and quantitative studies demonstrated the positive effects of physical exercise. An umbrella review in residential aged care settings corroborated these findings, highlighting the benefits of physical activities including dancing, walking, and body movements, performed with or without music [36]. In alignment with the outcomes related to music interventions, various strategies that involve dance therapy or movement synchronized with music showed reductions in agitation, aggression, anxiety, and wandering [36].

4.4.1.3 Personally Tailored Activities

Beyond the findings on music interventions, a Cochrane meta-analysis did not find sufficient evidence for sensory stimulation interventions [35]. Although evidence of a positive effect is limited, sensory stimulating interventions should still consider the personal interests and preferences of people with dementia. A review of 40 studies concluded that personalized interventions in residential aged care facilities can effectively improve mood, depression, and agitation [36]. Another review, a Cochrane review of five randomized trials, found that personally tailored activities provided by family caregivers at home may reduce challenging behavior and improve the quality of life for people with dementia [45].

To summarize, sensory stimulation, which can encompass music and exercise, stands as a plausible treatment strategy for challenging behavior. This is especially true when these interventions are tailored to accommodate the needs, interests, and preferences of individuals with dementia.

4.4.2 Interventions for Caregivers

An important working mechanism within personally tailored interventions for challenging behavior can involve the reduction of caregiver burden. Tailoring care to an individual's interests and personality, an essential feature of person-centered care, has been found to reduce stress and burnout in staff [36]. For example, decreasing caregivers' burden can be attributed to an increased sense of competence [45]. A review of 23 non-pharmacological interventions focused on caregivers, not restricted to long-term care facilities, showed effect sizes on challenging behavior at least equal to those of pharmacotherapy [46]. These interventions included elements that could increase a caregiver's sense of competence (e.g., skills training, education, activity planning, environmental modifications) and elements focused on caregiver well-being (e.g., provision of support and self-care interventions like health management and stress reduction). Interventions focused on caregivers were also evaluated in a recent meta-analysis of 22 high-quality studies showing decreased care burden and improved general health among family caregivers [12]. Notably, although multicomponent interventions showed larger effects on depression in family caregivers and seemed to improve general health more than psychoeducation alone, a single-component intervention with only psychoeducation appeared more effective at reducing care burden. Multicomponent interventions combine several conceptually different components such as psychoeducation, peer support, exercise, cognitive rehabilitation, pleasant activities, and occupational therapy. The larger effects of psychoeducation in some studies might be explained by a better understanding of the education needs of family carers [12]. A recent review on the needs of caregivers underscored that providing caregivers with information is a key area of support in dementia care [47].

To conclude, an approach that accommodates caregiver needs and preferences should definitely be considered alongside interventions that focus on the needs and preferences of people with dementia.

4.4.3 Environment and Green Care Elements

In accordance with the evidence discussed above, both professional and family caregivers—who form part of the social environment of people with dementia—are of great importance in reducing challenging behavior. Alongside the social environment, external variables pertaining to the physical environment should also be considered when addressing challenging behavior. Especially when considering sensory stimulation, it is crucial to consider that both indoor and outdoor environments are multisensory, involving light and sight, sound, smell, taste, and touch [48].

4.4.3.1 Built Environment

Three categories of interventions have been identified for built environments, namely those that involve (1) changing or redesigning existing physical space, (2) adding physical objects to an environment, and (3) changing the type of living environment [49]. People with dementia are sensitive to environmental stressors and cues. Therefore, the physical environment should match their cognitive abilities and functioning [50]. Based on 94 empirical studies and nine reviews in long-term care facilities, it can be argued that unit size, spatial layout, homelike character, sensory stimulation, and characteristics of social spaces affect challenging behavior and well-being in -residents. For example, smaller-scale common areas and more homelike or enhanced residential environments seem to improve mood and social interaction and reduce challenging behavior like aggression, agitation, and anxiety [50].

Although studies in long-term care do emphasize the importance of environmental attributes such as lighting, acoustics, room temperature, and the use of colors, contrast, and patterns [42], a recent Cochrane review concluded that evidence for the effects of environmental interventions on behavior is insufficient to draw clear conclusions [51]. It is difficult to differentiate the effects of the physical environment from those of other aspects of long-term care. Research on the physical environments of people with dementia living at home seems even more limited than research on long-term care facilities. Although it is argued that well-designed urban environments may reduce dementia risk through stimulation of social participation, proximity and accessibility, and recreation [52], it is unclear whether urban environments can affect or even cause challenging behavior. In contrast to many studies on physical environments in long-term care facilities, an extensive review showed only one study on the home environment that included a skill-improving intervention for family caregivers [53]. This intervention reduced both the caregiver burden and challenging behavior.

4.4.3.2 Green Care Elements

By introducing green spaces and natural elements into built neighborhood environments, elements of green care can be incorporated into both institutionalized or home care of people with dementia. Green care refers to a wide range of therapeutic interventions based on interactions with nature and animals. Studies have shown that engaging in outdoor activities (e.g., gardening) improves sleep and reduces stress, agitation, and aggressive behavior in dementia [50]. Alongside activities involving gardening care farming, and horticultural programs, green care may include recreational activities or activities guided by a professional with animals [54]. It has been advocated that green care elements and neighborhood environments with gardens, parks, and urban woodlands provide an avenue for meaningful activities, improve empowerment and positive risk-taking, and reinforce identity [55]. In natural environments, people with dementia report experiencing pleasure, relaxation, enjoyment of (the beauty of) nature, and being in fresh air. They enjoy observing wildlife and experiencing natural sounds and smells [56]. In addition, a review of 32 studies, although inconclusive, showed beneficial effects of animal-assisted therapy on challenging behavior [57].

4.4.3.3 Auditory Environment

There is growing recognition of the role of the auditory environment (sounds) in dementia care [42, 58]. Typically, long-term care facilities are characterized by high noise levels, which have been associated with increased challenging behavior like agitation and wandering [50]. During anti-pandemic COVID-19 measures, some nursing home residents showed a decrease in challenging behavior, which might have been caused by less noise and other changes in environmental stimuli [59]. However, sounds should not be considered solely in terms of noise, as some sounds can be meaningful and stimulate positive experiences [58]. A small study showed that introducing sounds such as the ocean, rain, wind, and running water can decrease agitated behavior [60]. This approach underlines the (positive) role of nature, even when attributes of nature are presented virtually.

To conclude, although more research is needed on the effects of physical and auditory environments on challenging behavior, adjustments in built and green environments need to be considered together with adjustments in sounds (soundscaping) or noise reduction.

4.4.4 Lifestyle Factors

There is limited research on the effects of lifestyle factors on challenging behavior. Research on preventing dementia and cognitive decline can be informative, as challenging behavior can be related to the progression of cognitive decline. Increasingly, evidence suggests that exercise, healthy nutrition, abstaining from or consuming very limited amounts of alcohol, maintaining social engagement, and having no history of smoking, hypertension, or sleep disturbances, may all be beneficial factors in preventing dementia and cognitive decline [61]. For example, a synthesis of 22 systematic reviews showed that multicomponent exercise might improve physical and cognitive functions and activities of daily living skills in dementia [62]. As already discussed, exercise can also decrease challenging behavior. Research on nutritional interventions, light interventions, and social engagement is briefly described below as other lifestyle factors.

4.4.4.1 Nutritional Interventions

Most people with dementia have a history of aberrant eating. Apathy, depression, memory loss, diet simplification, problems with biting, and inappropriate food practices by caregivers are associated with a decrease in the nutritional intake needed for a healthy brain [63, 64]. Some diets, such as the Mediterranean diet, Dietary Approaches to Stop Hypertension (DASH), and Nordic Prudent Dietary Pattern, are considered neuroprotective [61]. However, research on the effects of nutritional interventions on challenging behavior is very limited. For example, only four RCTs were identified in a meta-analysis by Haider et al. [65]. The meta-analysis demonstrated no significant effects on challenging behavior. Because the studies included were very heterogeneous in terms of the tested supplements—namely, a multicomponent nutritional supplement, an omega-3 supplement, and a supplement tailored to cognitive impairment—any generalization remains limited.

4.4.4.2 Light Interventions

A higher luminance level at the dining table might be effective for oral intake [42], which can contribute to healthy nutrition. Light can be considered as an attribute of the indoor environment. Light can also play a central role in the effects of outdoor activities. As previously discussed, outdoor activities are associated with less challenging behavior. This can be explained in part by bright day light. Adequate lighting may lead to decreased challenging behavior in general. Specifically, bright light therapy can improve quality of sleep, as was found in several studies [42].

4.4.4.3 Social Engagement

Studies in nursing home residents with dementia indicate that interventions facilitating meaningful interactions with others (i.e., social engagement) can be an effective alternative to medication use [66]. Reviews describe the effects of socially assistive robots on decreasing agitation and improving social interaction [67, 68], the effects of animal-assisted interventions on decreasing agitation/aggression and improving social behavior [57], and the effects of various virtual reality products that enhance social interaction [69]. Such reviews seem to support the hypothesis that social engagement in activity-based programs can explain beneficial effects on behavior in dementia [39]. Many activities include social engagement, even when real people are not present. Considering both the effects and the ease of implementation, it was argued that simulated presence therapy with video or audiotape recordings of family members is a useful strategy in nursing home practice to intervene in challenging behavior [43]. However, a Cochrane review on simulated presence did not find sufficient evidence of this [69].

To summarize, research on exercise, adequate lighting, and social engagement highlight the importance of these lifestyle factors. It is still not clear whether interventions that stimulate intake of healthy food can be used to treat challenging behavior. International initiatives such as World-Wide FINGERS [70] simultaneously combine diet, physical exercise, and cognitive training and reveal beneficial effects on cognitive functioning and the prevention of dementia. This suggests that multicomponent (or multidomain) interventions may also be prioritized for targeting challenging behavior. In real life, lifestyle factors do not occur in isolation, and they may interact or have a synergistic effect on different areas, including challenging behavior.

4.4.5 Psychotherapeutic Approaches

4.4.5.1 Psychotherapies

Research on so-called talk therapies based on the interaction between the individual with challenging behavior and the therapist (e.g., cognitive therapies or cognitive behavioral therapies) is limited. A review of non-pharmacological interventions in the residential aged care setting did not identify any relevant studies on these types of psychotherapies [36]. Two reviews on community-dwelling people with mild dementia showed that psychological treatment can be used to reduce depression and anxiety [71, 72]. A more recently published study on 200 people with mild cognitive impairment or early-stage dementia tested an intervention with elements from cognitive behavioral therapy, cognitive rehabilitation, and reminiscence therapy. The intervention did not show effects on challenging behavior measured with the NPI, but it did show reduced depressive symptoms [73].

As discussed in paragraph 4.2, reducing caregiver burden can also affect challenging behavior. A meta-analysis on cognitive behavioral therapies in family caregivers showed a reduction of subjective burden and depression in caregivers but no reduction of their anxiety or improved quality of life [74]. Another systematic review of psychological interventions involving both the family caregiver and the person with dementia (dyadic interventions) showed no effects on challenging behavior measured with the NPI, but it did show a reduction of anxiety and improvement of quality of life in people with dementia and, again, a reduction of family caregiver burden [75]. These results underscore the importance of the involvement of both halves of the dyad when delivering psychological interventions.

4.4.5.2 Reminiscence Therapy

Several publications have reviewed reminiscence therapy and interventions with reminiscence techniques, for example, as means to provide person-tailored, meaningful occupation, and cognitive interventions [36]. Precious memories therapy was successfully used in a large multidisciplinary trial aimed at depression in nursing homes [76]. The focus of this therapy is the recollection of specific positive memories from the main life periods of the person. Reminiscence techniques may use sensory stimulation like touch, taste, smell, and sound to help the patient remember or re-experience (mainly positive) emotionally loaded past events. Reminiscence interventions can be provided in individual sessions and group sessions. The latter may stimulate social engagement. A systematic review and meta-analysis showed that reminiscence interventions significantly reduce depression and challenging behavior in general and improve the quality of life for people with dementia [77]. In individuals without severe memory problems, life review therapy which includes recalling, evaluating, and reframing events, shows positive results on psychological well-being [78]. However, the conditions under which life review therapy can be applied in dementia care remain unclear. Difficulties interpreting and understanding verbal communication in psychotherapeutic sessions challenge the interaction between the therapist and the person with dementia. Evaluating and reframing can be too complex for people with dementia. Therefore, it is advised that precious memories therapy should focus on specific positive events [79].

4.4.5.3 Eye Movement Desensitization and Reprocessing (EMDR) On-the-Spot

EMDR is another therapy based on working with memories. EMDR is successfully used for treating post-traumatic stress disorder (PTSD) in different populations, and several studies support its effectiveness for the treatment of PTSD in very mild dementia [80]. A modified protocol for nursing home residents with dementia was successfully tested in Japan [80]. For this "on-the-spot EMDR method," a therapist obtains the patient's history from the chart and from the family. Simple basic words are used to communicate with people with dementia. Tapping a surface on both sides of the patient constitutes bilateral stimulation when restless challenging behavior appears. Results suggest that the protocol can be used for reducing challenging behavior related to a traumatic experience. However, further research is needed to understand whether and which modifications of EMDR are effective in addressing challenging behavior. The use of a standard EMDR protocol with the presence of a life partner was reported for a 69-year-old woman with mild dementia in the Netherlands [81].

Overall, while "talk therapies" may not always be feasible in dementia, certain forms of psychotherapeutic interventions can still be considered. Furthermore, it is important for professionals to consider involving or treating those who are in close contact with the person displaying challenging behavior. The following section provides more in-depth information on an approach that involves the participation of so-called mediators.

4.5 Mediative Therapy

Mediative therapy is a term used in the Netherlands to refer to treatments that involve individuals close to the patient. For individuals with dementia, these so-called mediators might include professional caregivers or family members. In other countries, this term corresponds with concepts such as behavioral approaches or behavioral modification as used in contexts like acquired brain injury [82, 83] as well as behavioral management in patients with psychiatric conditions [84] or dementia [85].

Mediative therapy might be indicated in the following circumstances: first, when the patient cannot benefit from direct interaction with a therapist due to severe cognitive problems; second, when the challenging behavior imposes a burden on individuals other than the patient; and third, when the challenging behavior is the result of social factors, such as issues with communication with professional or family caregivers, or specific triggers and activities [86, 87].

The methods of involving mediators can vary, ranging from providing consultations and advise [88] to offering guidance and support [89] and providing treatment that aims for change [86, 90, 91]. This section focuses specifically on treatment.

Several protocols for mediative therapy aimed at treating challenging behavior and incorporating elements of cognitive behavioral therapy have been described across various populations. These include children [92], individuals with mental disabilities [93], and older adults [94, 95].

A solution-oriented approach that concentrates on desired behavior complements the problem-oriented approach in mediative therapy. Examples of solution-oriented mediative therapy are described in works by Ferraz and Wellman [96], De Haan and Bannink [97], and Klaver [98]. In Klaver's protocol [86, 99], the problem-oriented approach, the solution-oriented approach, or a combination of both can be applied. The protocol combines Hermans et al.'s behavioral therapeutic step-by-step plan [100], a functional analysis outlined in a case study by Klaver and A-Tjak [87], and Bannink's solution-oriented vision on cognitive behavioral therapy [101]. The plan comprises six steps: problem identification, goal formulation, measurement, analyses, interventions, and evaluation.

Before embarking on mediative therapy, an analysis of behavior is conducted to understand potential causal relationships between variables that depict the patient's personal life story, personality, coping, and medical history. This is referred to as a case conceptualization [102]. Such an analysis can offer insights into the needs that shape the behavior or about elements in the patient's environment that influence the behavior. If an intervention based on this analysis is not possible, or if such an intervention does not yield improvements, the mediative protocol is subsequently initiated.

The first step of the mediative therapy protocol involves detailing the challenging behavior without interpretations (i.e., without using terms like "confused behavior" or "happy behavior"). For this purpose, questions can be utilized such as "what do you see someone doing or not doing when they are confused or happy?" or "what does this behavior look like?" If multiple behaviors are in play, it is crucial to explore whether they are interconnected. The manner in which behaviors can be related and what this implies for the treatment is described elsewhere [86, 99].

The second step, goal formulation, may include two goal types. The first type refers to changes in behavior such as reducing a challenging behavior, enhancing a desired behavior, or a combination of these two objectives. The second type pertains to improving the well-being of others with relation to the behavior being addressed;

for example, the goal can reduce the care team members' feelings of helplessness when repetitive calling occurs.

The third step of the described mediative therapy protocol consists of measuring the behavior. For this purpose, either an existing measurement scale (see above) or a custom-made instrument can be used (see Phase 1 of the cyclic approach).

The fourth step is functional analysis. This step involves three types of analyses (see Table 4.1). The first type provides insight into stimuli and situations that provoke challenging behavior and help maintain it. The second provides insight into the feelings, behaviors, and thoughts of others regarding the individual's behavior. The third aims to clarify which stimuli cause desired behavior and which stimuli help maintain it.

Step five of the protocol pertains to the interventions. The interventions are chosen based on functional analyses in step four. Table 4.1 outlines five intervention areas of focus (1 to 5). These intervention focal points are crucial for influencing the incidence and continuation of both challenging behavior (1, 2) and desired behavior (4, 5), as well as for improving the well-being of others (3). For points 1, 2, 4, & 5, behavioral interventions are necessary that identify the optimal strategies in relation to the patient's behavior. In contrast, for point 3, cognitive interventions are crucial for shifting the perception of others regarding their own well-being.

In the last step, step six, the effect of the interventions on the target variables is evaluated. The treatment can be concluded. However, if the effects are not satisfactory, the treatment cycle can be repeated, and step one is then re-started.

Research into mediative therapy shows positive effects on reducing challenging behavior [83]. In addition to primary effects, secondary effects are also described, such as the empowerment and emancipation of care teams in dealing with behavior [86]. Despite these benefits, there are some drawbacks. For example, mediative therapy is time-consuming, and the generalizability of personalized treatments is limited.

Table 4.1 Tree types of functional analyses with five intervention focus points

Challenging behavior		Desired behavior
Fa 1 patient	Fa 2 care team	Fa 3 patient
Situation (1)	Behavior patient	Situation (4)
	Feelings care team	
Behavior patient	Thoughts care team (3)	Behavior patient
	Behavior care team	
Consequences (2)	Consequences	Consequences (5)

Focus point 1 may concern noise in the living room that provokes a patient to scream. An environmental intervention can be employed to reduce this noise. Focus point 2 may concern the reaction of the care team to the screaming that, in turn, prompts the patient to scream more. An intervention may prescribe that the staff members provide unambiguous and limited attention to the patient's screaming. When screaming induces specific thoughts in the team members (focus point 3), which lead to feelings of powerlessness, a cognitive intervention can be utilized to address such thoughts and to mitigate such feelings. Playing music that calms the patient is an example of focus point 4. This calming effect can be reinforced by the care team through action point 5 by paying attention to this behavior.

4.6 Pharmacological Interventions

A crucial part of the analysis in phase 2 (*Prioritize and Analyze*) of the methodic cycle is a physical examination by a physician, as well as a review of the medications being used by the patient. For example, this could lead to a pharmacological treatment for pain using analgesics or the treatment of infections with antibiotics.

Physicians can be overwhelmed with the work involved in treating people with dementia and experience pressure from family caregivers and nursing home staff regarding the prescription of medication for challenging behavior [103]. However, recognition of the value of non-pharmacological strategies continues to grow [103].

Psychotropics are frequently used (20–70% of the time) for treating challenging behavior in people with dementia although a decline in their use has been observed over the last 15 years [104, 105]. However, psychotropics are regarded as a second choice in guidelines concerning the management of challenging behavior in people with dementia (see, for example, the 2018 NICE guideline [23]). This is based on their poor to moderate efficacy and considerable side effects, especially in people with brain disorders like dementia.

Box 4.1 provides a summary of the recommendations for the use of psychotropics for challenging behavior based on current evidence [23, 106–108].

Box 4.1 Recommendations for Pharmacological Interventions for Challenging Behavior

Agitation, Aggression, Distress, and Psychosis

Individuals with dementia experiencing symptoms of agitation, aggression, distress, and psychosis should only be treated with psychotropics as the first-line treatment if they are severely distressed/agitated or if there is an immediate risk of harm to the patient or others. If symptoms are less severe, non-pharmacological interventions (as detailed in paragraph 4) should be employed before considering a pharmacological intervention.

Haloperidol or risperidone may be considered for residents with Alzheimer's disease, vascular dementia, mixed dementias presenting symptoms of agitation, aggression, distress, and psychosis.

It is imperative to monitor effects and side effects (especially extrapyramidal features) diligently, and tapering/stopping is recommended after 3 months of use. However, in individuals with severe symptoms, this approach may not be successful.

For residents with Dementia with Lewy Bodies (DLB) or Parkinson's dementia, an acetylcholinesterase inhibitor is recommended, and clozapine can be used as a second option.

Depression and Anxiety

There appears to be insufficient supporting evidence for the effectiveness of antidepressants. Antidepressants should only be used in patients with severe depressive symptoms or a pre-existing severe depressive or anxiety disorder. Antidepressants with anticholinergic side effects should be avoided. In severe depression, electroconvulsive therapy can be considered.

For acute severe anxiety in residents with dementia, short acting benzodiazepines (lorazepam, oxazepam) may be used, but only for short-term periods (maximum of 4 weeks).

Sleep Problems

If non-pharmacological interventions prove ineffective for people with dementia experiencing severe sleep problems, melatonin, or trazodone (as a second choice) may be tried.

For other forms of challenging behavior in residents with dementia such as vocally disruptive behavior, wandering, resisting care, or sexually inappropriate behavior, there is no evidence for effectiveness of psychotropic drugs.

Note: Recommendations are based on guidelines and Cochrane reviews [23, 106–108].

4.7 Future Research and Implications for Practice

Unfortunately, research indicates that challenging behavior will not always disappear completely after treatment [14]. Some treatment strategies may have pervasive effects on outcomes other than those initially targeted (e.g., a pleasant activity plan intended to decrease depression in nursing home residents also showed effects on apathy [109]). Furthermore, although challenging behavior is associated with more rapid dementia progression, it is not clear whether interventions aimed at challenging behavior itself may slow dementia progression [13]. Therefore, it is important to monitor the effects of interventions on different outcomes, including those related to dementia progression.

In practice, many non-pharmacological interventions can be difficult to implement. Furthermore, pharmacological management of challenging behavior has often been seen as an ideal solution from the caregiver perspective, because it requires less involvement of others, including family and professional staff, compared to non-pharmacological interventions [110]. However, this does not mean that a pharmacological intervention must be chosen as the first treatment. Non-pharmacological interventions can be more effective or as effective as medication while side effects are mostly absent. Furthermore, some non-pharmacological interventions can be provided by family or integrated into the daily care activities of professional caregivers at a low cost. In this context, an educated and well-informed professional should be able to match an intervention to the person with dementia. Mediative therapy can be considered a promising and appropriate approach for choosing the right aims and strategies. However, further research is still needed on this method. Additionally, more research on multidomain interventions is required to understand whether and how multiple targeted aspects may result in a synergistic effect on the outcomes of interest.

Considering that non-pharmacological interventions include different components, it is often not clear which component is the most effective for which challenging behavior. Research on complex interventions may benefit from innovative designs that help facilitate understanding of what works for whom. In practice, professionals should use different strategies that may yield improvements in different areas of concern.

References

1. Borsje P, Wetzels RB, Lucassen PL, Pot AM, Koopmans RT. The course of neuropsychiatric symptoms in community-dwelling patients with dementia: a systematic review. Int Psychogeriatr. 2015;27(3):385–405. https://doi.org/10.1017/S1041610214002282.
2. Selbaek G, Engedal K, Benth JS, Bergh S. The course of neuropsychiatric symptoms in nursing-home patients with dementia over a 53-month follow-up period. Int Psychogeriatr. 2014;26(1):81–91. https://doi.org/10.1017/S1041610213001609.
3. de Oliveira AM, Radanovic M, de Mello PC, Buchain PC, Vizzotto AD, Celestino DL, Stella F, Piersol CV, Forlenza OV. Nonpharmacological interventions to reduce behavioral and psychological symptoms of dementia: a systematic review. Biomed Res Int. 2015;2015:218980. https://doi.org/10.1155/2015/218980.
4. van Duinen-van den IJssel IJCL, Mulders A, Smalbrugge M, Zwijsen SA, Appelhof B, Zuidema SU, de Vugt ME, Verhey FRJ, Bakker C, Koopmans R. Nursing staff distress associated with neuropsychiatric symptoms in young-onset dementia and late-onset dementia. J Am Med Dir Assoc. 2018;19(7):627–32. https://doi.org/10.1016/j.jamda.2017.10.004.
5. Kales HC, Gitlin LN, Lyketsos CG. Assessment and management of behavioral and psychological symptoms of dementia. BMJ. 2015;350:h369. https://doi.org/10.1136/bmj.h369.
6. Chan DC, Kasper JD, Black BS, Rabins PV. Prevalence and correlates of behavioral and psychiatric symptoms in community-dwelling elders with dementia or mild cognitive impairment: the Memory and Medical Care Study. Int J Geriatr Psychiatry. 2003;18(2):174–82. https://doi.org/10.1002/gps.781.
7. Kazui H, Yoshiyama K, Kanemoto H, Suzuki Y, Sato S, Hashimoto M, Ikeda M, Tanaka H, Hatada Y, Matsushita M, Nishio Y, Mori E, Tanimukai S, Komori K, Yoshida T, Shimizu H, Matsumoto T, Mori T, Kashibayashi T, Yokoyama K, Shimomura T, Kabeshita Y, Adachi H, Tanaka T. Differences of behavioral and psychological symptoms of dementia in disease severity in four major dementias. PLoS One. 2016;11(8):e0161092. https://doi.org/10.1371/journal.pone.0161092.
8. Selbaek G, Engedal K, Bergh S. The prevalence and course of neuropsychiatric symptoms in nursing home patients with dementia: a systematic review. J Am Med Dir Assoc. 2013;14(3):161–9. https://doi.org/10.1016/j.jamda.2012.09.027.
9. Bransvik V, Granvik E, Minthon L, Nordstrom P, Nagga K. Mortality in patients with behavioural and psychological symptoms of dementia: a registry-based study. Aging Ment Health. 2021;25(6):1101–9. https://doi.org/10.1080/13607863.2020.1727848.
10. Ornstein K, Gaugler JE. The problem with "problem behaviors": a systematic review of the association between individual patient behavioral and psychological symptoms and caregiver depression and burden within the dementia patient–caregiver dyad. Int Psychogeriatr. 2012; 24(10):1536–52. https://doi.org/10.1017/S1041610212000737.

11. Braun A, Trivedi DP, Dickinson A, Hamilton L, Goodman C, Gage H, Manthorpe J. Managing behavioural and psychological symptoms in community dwelling older people with dementia: 2. A systematic review of qualitative studies. Dementia. 2019;18(7–8):2950–70. https://doi.org/10.1177/1471301218762856.
12. Teahan A, Lafferty A, McAuliffe E, Phelan A, O'Sullivan L, O'Shea D, Nicholson E, Fealy G. Psychosocial interventions for family carers of people with dementia: a systematic review and meta-analysis. J Aging Health. 2020;32(9):1198–213. https://doi.org/10.1177/0898264319899793.
13. Preuss UW, Wong JW, Koller G. Treatment of behavioral and psychological symptoms of dementia: a systematic review. Psychiatr Pol. 2016;50(4):679–715. https://doi.org/10.12740/PP/64477. (Przeglad metod leczenia behawioralnych i psychologicznych symptomow otepienia (BPSD).)
14. Tible OP, Riese F, Savaskan E, von Gunten A. Best practice in the management of behavioural and psychological symptoms of dementia. Ther Adv Neurol Disord. 2017;10(8):297–309. https://doi.org/10.1177/1756285617712979.
15. IPA. The IPA Complete Guides to Behavioral and Psychological Symptoms of Dementia (BPSD); 2015.
16. Gerlach LB, Kales HC. Managing behavioral and psychological symptoms of dementia. Psychiatr Clin North Am. 2018;41(1):127–39. https://doi.org/10.1016/j.psc.2017.10.010.
17. Gerritsen DL, Smalbrugge M, Veldwijk-Rouwenhorst AE, Wetzels R, Zuidema SU, Koopmans R. The difficulty with studying challenging behavior. J Am Med Dir Assoc. 2019;20(7):879–81. https://doi.org/10.1016/j.jamda.2019.01.148.
18. Cohen-Mansfield. Theoretical frameworks for behavioral problems in dementia. Alzheim Care Q. 2000;1(4):8–21.
19. Hall GR, Buckwalter KC. Progressively lowered stress threshold: a conceptual model for care of adults with Alzheimer's disease. Arch Psychiatr Nurs. 1987;1(6):399–406. https://www.ncbi.nlm.nih.gov/pubmed/3426250.
20. Droes RM. Insight in coping with dementia: listening to the voice of those who suffer from it. Aging Ment Health. 2007;11(2):115–8. https://doi.org/10.1080/13607860601154658.
21. Dröes RMI. In Beweging, over psychosociale hulpverlening aan demente ouderen. [In Movement, on psychosocial care for older people with dementia], Academic thesis. VU University; 1991.
22. Richards KC, Beck CK. Progressively lowered stress threshold model: understanding behavioral symptoms of dementia. J Am Geriatr Soc. 2004;52(10):1774–5.
23. NICE. Dementia: assessment, management and support for people living with dementia and their carers (NG97). National Institute for Health and Care Excellence; 2018.
24. NHS. Guidelines for the management of Behavioural and Psychological Symptoms of Dementia (BPSD); 2019.
25. Verenso. Probleemgedrag bij mensen met dementie. Vereniging van specialisten ouderengeneeskunde—Nederlands Instituut voor Psychologen; 2018.
26. Zwijsen SA, Smalbrugge M, Eefsting JA, Gerritsen DL, Hertogh CM, Pot AM. Grip on challenging behavior: process evaluation of the implementation of a care program. Trials. 2014;15:302. https://doi.org/10.1186/1745-6215-15-302.
27. Lichtwarck B, Selbaek G, Kirkevold O, Rokstad AM, Benth JS, Myhre J, Nybakken S, Bergh S. TIME—Targeted interdisciplinary model for evaluation and treatment of neuropsychiatric symptoms: protocol for an effectiveness-implementation cluster randomized hybrid trial. BMC Psychiatry. 2016;16:233. https://doi.org/10.1186/s12888-016-0944-0.
28. Cummings JL, Mega M, Gray K, Rosenberg-Thompson S, Carusi DA, Gornbein J. The neuropsychiatric inventory: comprehensive assessment of psychopathology in dementia. Neurology. 1994;44(12):2308–14. http://www.ncbi.nlm.nih.gov/entrez/query.fcgi?cmd=Retrieve&db=PubMed&dopt=Citation&list_uids=7991117.
29. Reisberg B, Monteiro I, Torossian C, Auer S, Shulman MB, Ghimire S, Boksay I, Guillo BenArous F, Osorio R, Vengassery A, Imran S, Shaker H, Noor S, Naqvi S, Kenowsky S, Xu J. The BEHAVE-AD assessment system: a perspective, a commentary on new findings,

and a historical review. Dement Geriatr Cogn Disord. 2014;38(1–2):89–146. https://doi.org/10.1159/000357839.

30. Marin RS, Biedrzycki RC, Firinciogullari S. Reliability and validity of the Apathy Evaluation Scale. Psychiatry Res. 1991;38(2):143–62. http://www.ncbi.nlm.nih.gov/entrez/query.fcgi?cmd=Retrieve&db=PubMed&dopt=Citation&list_uids=1754629.
31. Alexopoulos GS, Abrams RC, Young RC, Shamoian CA. Cornell scale for depression in dementia. Biol Psychiatry. 1988;23(3):271–84. https://doi.org/10.1016/0006-3223(88)90038-8.
32. Cohen-Mansfield J. Instruction manual for the Cohen-Mansfield Agitation Inventory (CMAI). The Research Institute of the Hebrew Home of Greater Washington; 1991.
33. Leontjevas R, Teerenstra S, Smalbrugge M, Koopmans RT, Gerritsen DL. Quality of life assessments in nursing homes revealed a tendency of proxies to moderate patients' self-reports. J Clin Epidemiol. 2016;80:123–33. https://doi.org/10.1016/j.jclinepi.2016.07.009.
34. Cloak N, Al Khalili Y. Behavioral and psychological symptoms in dementia. In: StatPearls. Treasure Island: StatPearls Publishing; 2023. https://www.ncbi.nlm.nih.gov/pubmed/31855379.
35. Dyer SM, Harrison SL, Laver K, Whitehead C, Crotty M. An overview of systematic reviews of pharmacological and non-pharmacological interventions for the treatment of behavioral and psychological symptoms of dementia. Int Psychogeriatr. 2018;30(3):295–309. https://doi.org/10.1017/S1041610217002344.
36. Koch J, Amos JG, Beattie E, Lautenschlager NT, Doyle C, Anstey KJ, Mortby ME. Non-pharmacological interventions for neuropsychiatric symptoms of dementia in residential aged care settings: an umbrella review. Int J Nurs Stud. 2022;128:104187. https://doi.org/10.1016/j.ijnurstu.2022.104187.
37. Chenoweth L, Stein-Parbury J, Lapkin S, Wang A, Liu Z, Williams A. Effects of person-centered care at the organisational-level for people with dementia. A systematic review. PLoS One. 2019;14(2):e0212686. https://doi.org/10.1371/journal.pone.0212686.
38. Lee KH, Lee JY, Kim B. Person-centered care in persons living with dementia: a systematic review and meta-analysis. Gerontologist. 2022;62(4):e253–64. https://doi.org/10.1093/geront/gnaa207.
39. Knippenberg IAH, Reijnders J, Gerritsen DL, Leontjevas R. The association between specific activity components and depression in nursing home residents: the importance of the social component. Aging Ment Health. 2021:1–8. https://doi.org/10.1080/13607863.2019.1671312.
40. Knippenberg IAH, Leontjevas R, Declercq I, De Vriendt P, Persoon A, Verboon P, van Lankveld JJDM, Gerritsen DL. Actions to Improve Mood (AIM): Vragenlijsten over stemmingsbevorderende handelingen in verpleeghuizen en woonzorgcentra. [Poster] SANO Wetenschapsdag, Oegstgeest, Netherlands; 2022.
41. Alm AK, Danielsson S, Porskrog-Kristiansen L. Non-pharmalogical interventions towards behavioural and psychological symptoms of dementia—an integrated literature review. Open J Nurs. 2018;8:434–47.
42. Marquardt G, Bueter K, Motzek T. Impact of the design of the built environment on people with dementia: an evidence-based review. HERD. 2014;8(1):127–57. https://doi.org/10.1177/193758671400800111.
43. Meyer C, O'Keefe F. Non-pharmacological interventions for people with dementia: a review of reviews. Dementia (London). 2020;19(6):1927–54. https://doi.org/10.1177/1471301218813234.
44. https://pubmed.ncbi.nlm.nih.gov/37768499/.
45. Mohler R, Renom A, Renom H, Meyer G. Personally tailored activities for improving psychosocial outcomes for people with dementia in community settings. Cochrane Database Syst Rev. 2020;8(8):CD010515. https://doi.org/10.1002/14651858.CD010515.pub2.
46. Brodaty H, Burns K. Nonpharmacological management of apathy in dementia: a systematic review [Review]. Am J Geriatr Psychiatry. 2012;20(7):549–64. https://doi.org/10.1097/JGP.0b013e31822be242.

47. Queluz F, Kervin E, Wozney L, Fancey P, McGrath PJ, Keefe J. Understanding the needs of caregivers of persons with dementia: a scoping review. Int Psychogeriatr. 2020;32(1):35–52. https://doi.org/10.1017/S1041610219000243.
48. Gan DRY, Chaudhury H, Mann J, Wister AV. Dementia-friendly neighborhood and the built environment: a scoping review. Gerontologist. 2022;62(6):e340–56. https://doi.org/10.1093/geront/gnab019.
49. Soril LJ, Leggett LE, Lorenzetti DL, Silvius J, Robertson D, Mansell L, Holroyd-Leduc J, Noseworthy TW, Clement FM. Effective use of the built environment to manage behavioural and psychological symptoms of dementia: a systematic review. PLoS One. 2014;9(12):e115425. https://doi.org/10.1371/journal.pone.0115425.
50. Chaudhury H, Cooke HA, Cowie H, Razaghi L. The influence of the physical environment on residents with dementia in long-term care settings: a review of the empirical literature. Gerontologist. 2018;58(5):e325–37. https://doi.org/10.1093/geront/gnw259.
51. Harrison SL, Dyer SM, Laver KE, Milte RK, Fleming R, Crotty M. Physical environmental designs in residential care to improve quality of life of older people. Cochrane Database Syst Rev. 2022;3(3):CD012892. https://doi.org/10.1002/14651858.CD012892.pub2.
52. Rohr S, Rodriguez FS, Siemensmeyer R, Muller F, Romero-Ortuno R, Riedel-Heller SG. How can urban environments support dementia risk reduction? A qualitative study. Int J Geriatr Psychiatry. 2022;37(1) https://doi.org/10.1002/gps.5626.
53. Trivedi DP, Braun A, Dickinson A, Gage H, Hamilton L, Goodman C, Ashaye K, Iliffe S, Manthorpe J. Managing behavioural and psychological symptoms in community dwelling older people with dementia: 1. A systematic review of the effectiveness of interventions. Dementia (London). 2019;18(7–8):2925–49. https://doi.org/10.1177/1471301218762851.
54. Sempik J, Hine R, Wilcox D. Green care: a conceptual framework, A report of the Working Group on the Health Benefits of Green Care, COST Action 866, Green Care in Agriculture. Centre for Child and Family Research, Loughborough University; 2010.
55. Mmako NJ, Courtney-Pratt H, Marsh P. Green spaces, dementia and a meaningful life in the community: a mixed studies review. Health Place. 2020;63:102344. https://doi.org/10.1016/j.healthplace.2020.102344.
56. Barrett J, Evans S, Mapes N. Green dementia care in accommodation and care settings: a literature review. Housing Care Support. 2019;22(4):193–206.
57. Yakimicki ML, Edwards NE, Richards E, Beck AM. Animal-assisted intervention and dementia: a systematic review. Clin Nurs Res. 2019;28(1):9–29. https://doi.org/10.1177/1054773818756987.
58. Leontjevas R. Soundscape in nursing homes as a treatment strategy for challenging behavior in dementia? Int Psychogeriatr. 2021;33(6):553–6. https://doi.org/10.1017/S1041610220003348.
59. Knippenberg IAH, Leontjevas R, Nijsten JMH, Bakker C, Koopmans R, Gerritsen DL. Stimuli changes and challenging behavior in nursing homes during the COVID-19 pandemic. BMC Geriatr. 2022;22(1):142. https://doi.org/10.1186/s12877-022-02824-y.
60. Lin LW, Weng SC, Wu HS, Tsai LJ, Lin YL, Yeh SH. The effects of white noise on agitated behaviors, mental status, and activities of daily living in older adults with dementia. J Nurs Res. 2018;26(1):2–9. https://doi.org/10.1097/JNR.0000000000000211.
61. Dominguez LJ, Veronese N, Vernuccio L, Catanese G, Inzerillo F, Salemi G, Barbagallo M. Nutrition, physical activity, and other lifestyle factors in the prevention of cognitive decline and dementia. Nutrients. 2021;13:4080.
62. McDermott O, Charlesworth G, Hogervorst E, Stoner C, Moniz-Cook E, Spector A, Csipke E, Orrell M. Psychosocial interventions for people with dementia: a synthesis of systematic reviews. Aging Ment Health. 2019;23(4):393–403. https://doi.org/10.1080/13607863.2017.1423031.

63. Bianchi VE, Herrera PF, Laura R. Effect of nutrition on neurodegenerative diseases. A systematic review. Nutr Neurosci. 2021;24(10):810–34. https://doi.org/10.1080/1028415X.2019.1681088.
64. Cipriani G, Carlesi C, Lucetti C, Danti S, Nuti A. v. Am J Alzheimers Dis Other Dement. 2016;31(8):706–16. https://doi.org/10.1177/1533317516673155.
65. Haider S, Schwarzinger A, Stefanac S, Soysal P, Smith L, Veronese N, Dorner TE, Grabovac I. Nutritional supplements for neuropsychiatric symptoms in people with dementia: a systematic review and meta-analysis. Int J Geriatr Psychiatry. 2020;35(11):1285–91. https://doi.org/10.1002/gps.5407.
66. Saleh N, Penning M, Cloutier D, Mallidou A, Nuernberger K, Taylor D. Social engagement and antipsychotic use in addressing the behavioral and psychological symptoms of dementia in long-term care facilities. Can J Nurs Res. 2017;49(4):144–52. https://doi.org/10.1177/0844562117726253.
67. Ong YC, Tang A, Tam W. Effectiveness of robot therapy in the management of behavioural and psychological symptoms for individuals with dementia: a systematic review and meta-analysis. J Psychiatr Res. 2021;140:381–94. https://doi.org/10.1016/j.jpsychires.2021.05.077.
68. Yamazaki R, Kase H, Nishio S, Ishiguro H. A conversational robotic approach to dementia symptoms. In: Proceedings of the 7th International Conference on Human-Agent Interaction (HAI'19). Kyoto, Japan, 2019; p. 8.
69. Appel L, Ali S, Narag T, Mozeson K, Pasat Z, Orchanian-Cheff A, Campos JL. Virtual reality to promote wellbeing in persons with dementia: a scoping review. J Rehabil Assist Technol Eng. 2021;8:20556683211053952. https://doi.org/10.1177/20556683211053952.
70. Rosenberg A, Mangialasche F, Ngandu T, Solomon A, Kivipelto M. Multidomain interventions to prevent cognitive impairment, Alzheimer's disease, and dementia: From FINGER to World-Wide FINGERS. J Prev Alzheimers Dis. 2020;7:29–36. https://doi.org/10.14283/jpad.2019.41.
71. Cheston R, Ivanecka A. Individual and group psychotherapy with people diagnosed with dementia: a systematic review of the literature. Int J Geriatr Psychiatry. 2017;32(1):3–31. https://doi.org/10.1002/gps.4529.
72. Orgeta V, Qazi A, Spector A, Orrell M. Psychological treatments for depression and anxiety in dementia and mild cognitive impairment: systematic review and meta-analysis. Br J Psychiatry. 2015;207(4):293–8. https://doi.org/10.1192/bjp.bp.114.148130.
73. Tonga JB, Saltyte Benth J, Arnevik EA, Werheid K, Korsnes MS, Ulstein ID. Managing depressive symptoms in people with mild cognitive impairment and mild dementia with a multicomponent psychotherapy intervention: a randomized controlled trial. Int Psychogeriatr. 2021;33(3):217–31. https://doi.org/10.1017/S1041610220000216.
74. Verreault P, Turcotte V, Ouellet MC, Robichaud LA, Hudon C. Efficacy of cognitive-behavioural therapy interventions on reducing burden for caregivers of older adults with a neurocognitive disorder: a systematic review and meta-analysis. Cogn Behav Ther. 2021;50(1):19–46. https://doi.org/10.1080/16506073.2020.1819867.
75. Poon E. A systematic review and meta-analysis of dyadic psychological interventions for BPSD, quality of life and/or caregiver burden in dementia or MCI. Clin Gerontol. 2022;45(4):777–97. https://doi.org/10.1080/07317115.2019.1694117.
76. Leontjevas R, Gerritsen DL, Smalbrugge M, Teerenstra S, Vernooij-Dassen MJ, Koopmans RT. A structural multidisciplinary approach to depression management in nursing-home residents: a multicentre, stepped-wedge cluster-randomised trial. Lancet. 2013;381(9885):2255–64. https://doi.org/10.1016/S0140-6736(13)60590-5.
77. Park K, Lee S, Yang J, Song T, Hong GS. A systematic review and meta-analysis on the effect of reminiscence therapy for people with dementia. Int Psychogeriatr. 2019;31(11):1581–97. https://doi.org/10.1017/S1041610218002168.

78. Tam W, Poon SN, Mahendran R, Kua EH, Wu XV. The effectiveness of reminiscence-based intervention on improving psychological well-being in cognitively intact older adults: a systematic review and meta-analysis. Int J Nurs Stud. 2021;114:103847. https://doi.org/10.1016/j.ijnurstu.2020.103847.
79. van Venrooij I, Spijker J, Westerhof GJ, Leontjevas R, Gerritsen DL. Applying intervention mapping to improve the applicability of precious memories, an intervention for depressive symptoms in nursing home residents. Int J Environ Res Public Health. 2019;16(24) https://doi.org/10.3390/ijerph16245163.
80. Amano T, Toichi M. Effectiveness of the on-the-spot-EMDR method for the treatment of behavioral symptoms in patients with severe dementia. J EMDR Pract Res. 2014;8(2) https://doi.org/10.1891/1933-3196.8.2.50.
81. van der Wielen M, Robben H, Mark RE. The applicability and effect of EMDR in a patient with a mild stage of Alzheimer's disease. J EMDR Pract Res. 2019;13(1):51–60.
82. Alderman N, Knight C, Henman C. Aggressive behaviour observed within a neurobehavioural rehabilitation service: utility of the OAS-MNR in clinical audit and applied research. Brain Inj. 2002;16(6):469–89. https://doi.org/10.1080/02699050110118458.
83. Alderman N, Wood RL. Neurobehavioural approaches to the rehabilitation of challenging behaviour. NeuroRehabilitation. 2013;32(4):761–70. https://doi.org/10.3233/NRE-130900.
84. Rewilak D. Behavior management strategies. In: Conn DK, Hermann N, Kaye A, Rewilak D, Schogt B, editors. Practical psychiatry in the long term care facility. A handbook for staff. Boston, MA: Hogrefe & Huber; 2001. p. 199–221.
85. Moniz Cook ED, Swift K, James I, Malouf R, De Vugt M, Verhey F. Functional analysis-based interventions for challenging behaviour in dementia. Cochrane Database Syst Rev. 2012;(2):CD006929. https://doi.org/10.1002/14651858.CD006929.pub2.
86. Klaver MG. Mediatieve therapie. In: Smits P, Ponds R, Farenhorst N, Klaver MG, Verbeek R. Handboek neuropsychotherapie. Boom; 2016.
87. Klaver MG, A-Tjak J. Mediatieve gedragstherapie in het verpleeghuis: Het gebruik van cognitief gedragstherapeutische analyses en cognitieve interventies met een zorgteam. Gedragstherapie. 2006;39:5–21.
88. Tharp R, Wetzel R. Behavior modification in the natural environment. Cambridge, MA: Academic Press; 1969.
89. Allewijn M, Haaring L. Teambegeleiding. In: Vink M, Kuin Y, Westerhof G, Lamers S (red.), Handboek ouderenpsychologie; 2017.
90. Geelen R, Bleijenberg G. Proef op de som. Illustratie van gedragstherapie in het psychogeriatrische verpleeghuis. Gedragstherapie. 1999;32:79–104.
91. Hamer AFM. Veranderen via een omweg: Mediatieve therapie. In: Vink MT, Broek P (red.), Oud geleerd, oud gedaan: Gedragstherapie bij ouderen. Uitgaven serie Psychologie en ouderen deel 3. Bohn Stafleu van Loghum; 1998.
92. Bosch JD, Ringrose HJ. Mediatietherapie met ouders: individueel en in groepen. Praktijkreeks Gedragstherapie; 1997..
93. Raemdonck K. Mediatietherapie in de residentiële zorg voor kinderen en jeugdigen Garant; 2009.
94. Cohn MD, Smyer MA, Horgas AL. The ABC's of behavior change: skills for working with behavior problems in nursing homes. Alberta: Venture Publishing; 1994.
95. James, I. A. (2013). Cognitieve gedragstherapie voor ouderen. Een praktische gids voor hulpverleners. LannooCampus.
96. Ferraz H, Wellman N. The integration of solution-focused brief therapy principles in nursing: a literature review. J Psychiatr Ment Health Nurs. 2008;15(1):37–44. https://doi.org/10.1111/j.1365-2850.2007.01204.x.
97. de Haan R, Bannink FP. Oplossingsgerichte therapie met ouderen; 2019.
98. Klaver MG. Omgaan met (probleem)gedrag in het verpleeghuis. Een mediatieve inzet van positieve psychologie en oplossingsgerichte therapie. Tijdschrift voor Positieve Psychol. 2020;5(2):23–8.

99. Klaver MG. Protocol voor het mediatief toepassen van cognitieve gedragstherapie met een zorgteam; 2017. www.neuropsychologischebehandeling.nl.
100. Hermans D, Raes F, Orlemans E. Inleiding tot de gedragstherapie. Houten: Bohn Stafleu van Loghum; 2018.
101. Bannink FP. Oplossingsgerichte vragen: handboek oplossingsgerichte gespreksvoering. San Diego: Harcourt; 2013.
102. Korrelboom K, ten Broeke E. Geïntegreerde cognitieve gedragstherapie: Handboek voor theorie en praktijk. Coutinho; 2019.
103. Jennings AA, Foley T, Walsh KA, Coffey A, Browne JP, Bradley CP. General practitioners' knowledge, attitudes and experiences of managing behavioural and psychological symptoms of dementia: protocol of a mixed methods systematic review and meta-ethnography. Syst Rev. 2018;7(1):62. https://doi.org/10.1186/s13643-018-0732-7.
104. Du J, Janus S, Voorthuis B, van Manen J, Achterberg W, Smalbrugge M, Zwijsen S, Gerritsen D, Koopmans R, Zuidema S. Time trends in psychotropic drug prescriptions in Dutch nursing home residents with dementia between 2003 and 2018. Int J Geriatr Psychiatry. 2022;37(4) https://doi.org/10.1002/gps.5697.
105. Janus SI, van Manen JG, IJzerman MJ, Zuidema SU. Psychotropic drug prescriptions in Western European nursing homes. Int Psychogeriatr. 2016;28(11):1775–90. https://doi.org/10.1017/S1041610216001150.
106. Dudas R, Malouf R, McCleery J, Dening T. Antidepressants for treating depression in dementia. Cochrane Database Syst Rev. 2018;8(8):CD003944. https://doi.org/10.1002/14651858.CD003944.pub2.
107. McCleery J, Sharpley AL. Pharmacotherapies for sleep disturbances in dementia. Cochrane Database Syst Rev. 2020;11(11):CD009178. https://doi.org/10.1002/14651858.CD009178.pub4.
108. Van Leeuwen E, Petrovic M, van Driel ML, De Sutter AI, Vander Stichele R, Declercq T, Christiaens T. Withdrawal versus continuation of long-term antipsychotic drug use for behavioural and psychological symptoms in older people with dementia. Cochrane Database Syst Rev. 2018;3(3):CD007726. https://doi.org/10.1002/14651858.CD007726.pub3.
109. Leontjevas R, Teerenstra S, Smalbrugge M, Vernooij-Dassen MJ, Bohlmeijer ET, Gerritsen DL, Koopmans RT. More insight into the concept of apathy: a multidisciplinary depression management program has different effects on depressive symptoms and apathy in nursing homes [Research Support, Non-U.S. Gov't]. Int Psychogeriatr. 2013;25(12):1941–52. https://doi.org/10.1017/S1041610213001440.
110. Magierski R, Sobow T, Schwertner E, Religa D. Pharmacotherapy of behavioral and psychological symptoms of dementia: state of the art and future progress. Front Pharmacol. 2020;11:1168. https://doi.org/10.3389/fphar.2020.01168.

General Considerations on Psychopharmacology in Older People

5

Therapeutic Conflicts with Benzodiazepines and Z-drugs

Jorge Juri, Alejandro Serra, and Dante Boveris

5.1 Background

We need to know the importance of existing knowledge about the risk of falls associated with benzodiazepines (BZDs) and Z-drugs in older people with an emphasis on proper prescribing.

Falls are, after road traffic injuries, the second leading cause of trauma-related death worldwide.

Approximately 28–35% of people aged of 65 and over fall each year, increasing to 32–42% for those over 70 years of age. The frequency of falls increases with age and frailty level. Older people who are living in nursing homes fall more often than those who are living in community. Approximately 30–50% of people living in long-term care institutions fall each year, and 40% of them experienced recurrent falls. Falls lead to 20–30% of mild to severe injuries and are the underlying cause of 10–15% of all emergency department visits [1].

In Western Europe, 54,504 older adults died due to falls in 2017 [2].

Falls in older people are often associated with serious injuries, predominantly hip fractures. Falls lead to more than 50% of injury-related hospitalizations among people over 65 years and older. The major underlying causes for fall-related hospital admission are hip fracture, traumatic brain injuries, and upper limb injuries. To add insult to injury, falls lead to hospital stays of 7–20 days with subsequent deep vein thrombosis and pressure ulcers risk due to patient immobility [1].

J. Juri (✉)
University of Business and Social Sciences, Buenos Aires, Argentina

A. Serra
Department of Pharmacology, School of Medicine, University of Buenos Aires (UBA) School of Medicine, University of Buenos Aires, Buenos Aires, Argentina

D. Boveris
Vicente Lopez Private Institute, Buenos Aires, Argentina

N. Veronese, A. Marseglia (eds.), *Psychogeriatrics*, Practical Issues in Geriatrics,
https://doi.org/10.1007/978-3-031-58488-6_5

In addition, falls can lead to loss of independence, loss of self-confidence (post-fall syndrome), increased risk of institutionalization, and decreased quality of life [3, 4].

We can say that one of the most prominent and modifiable risk factors is the use of drugs that increase the risk of falls [5, 6].

Fall prevention guidelines recommend a medication review to identify inappropriate use of FRID "(Fall-risk increading drug)" as part of the multi-design fall prevention strategy [7].

In 2020, a group of European experts developed the STOPP Fall tool, a specific detection tool that helps deprescribing in older adults at high risk of falling.

This tool was created using a Delphi expert consensus process and consists of 14 classes of drugs [6].

A cross-sectional study including 107,504 adults aged 65 years and over from their first admission to two academic hospitals from 2010 to 2018 in West Virginia, U.S. reveals that 13.5% were using benzodiazepines at home [8].

The prevalence of BZD use among Dutch nursing home residents is 39.2%. Continuous use accounts for 22.9%, and only-as-needed use accounts for 16.3% [9].

Some risk factors cannot be changed (demography, diseases), others are potentially modifiable (health and functional status, including FRID) (Fig. 5.1).

A prospective cohort study showed that patients using long-acting diazepam were three times more likely to have a drop in the previous 90 days compared to non-users and all other BZD users. Daytime sedation is also more likely manifested with longer half-life BZD than with shorter half-life BZD.

On the other hand, zolpidem significantly increased the risk of falls in hospitalized patients [11] (Fig. 5.2).

Several studies also reported an effect of dose dependency on the risk of falls. Doses of BZD >1 mg/day in diazepam equivalents were significantly associated with falls among hospitalized older people (Fig. 5.3).

5.2 Relationship with Delirium

The reported prevalence of delirium among hospitalized older patients ranges from 14% to 56%, and nearly one-third appears to be drug-induced [12].

The use of potentially inappropriate medications in older people strongly discourages prolonged BZDs in older people due to the increased risk of confusion, delirium, falls, fractures, and car accidents.

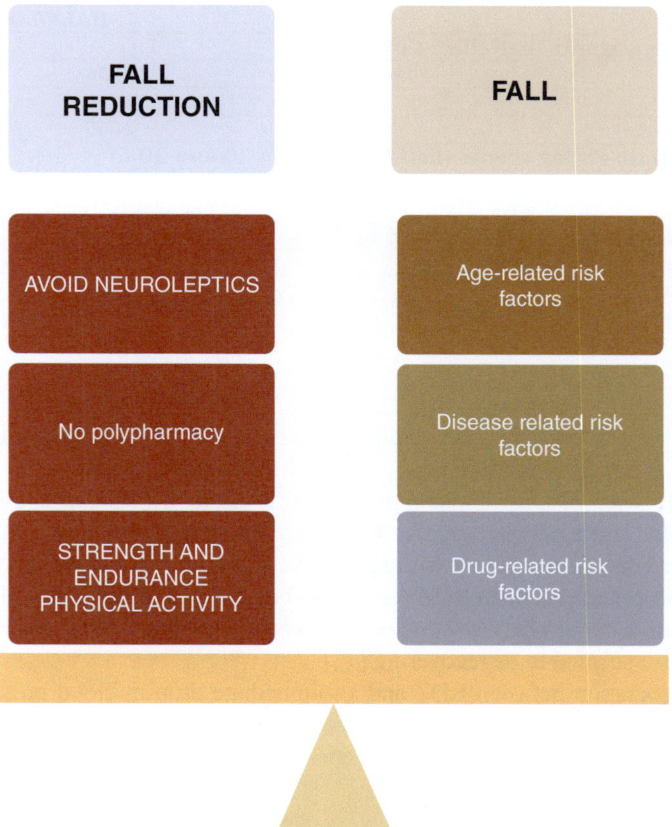

Fig. 5.1 Risk balance. This balance indicates the probability that an older adult has of falling according to the predominance of one column or another [10]

Z-drug	T_{max} (h)	Oral bioavailability	Elimination $t_{½}$ (h)	Dose range	Metabolism
Zolpidem IR	1–2	65–70 %	2.5–3	5–10 mg	*CYP 3A4, 2C9,* 1A2
Zolpidem ER	1.5–2.5	65–70 %	2.5–3	6.25–12.5 mg	
Zopiclone	1.5–2	75–80 %	5–6	3.75–7.5 mg	*CYP 3A4*, 2C8
Eszopiclone	1–1.5	75–80 %	6–7	1–3 mg	*CYP 3A4*, 2E1
Zaleplon	0.7–1.4	30 %	~1	5–20 mg	*Aldehyde oxidase*, CYP 3A4

Fig. 5.2 Elimination half-life of BZDs and Z-drugs

5.3 Effects on Orthostatic Hypotension and Postural Instability

Orthostatic Hypotension (OH) is defined as a reduction in SBP of at least 20 mmHg or DBP of at least 10 mmHg within 3 min of standing from the supine position or a

	HALF-LIFE (hours)
Long-acting agents (half-life > 20h)	
Clobazam	36
Diazepam	48
Flunitrazepam	24-60
Intermediate-acting agents (half-life between 10 and 20 h)	
Alprazolam	12-15
Lorazepam	12-16
Short-acting agents (half-life < 10 h)	
Oxazepam	6-8
Zolpidem	2-4
Zopiclone	5

Fig. 5.3 Half-life of action of benzodiazepines [10]

similar drop in blood pressure within 3 min of the vertical tilting table test by at least 60°.

A study with 538 participants and 33 BZD users with mean age 72.7 years reported that older people who use BZD have an increased risk of OH due to an exaggerated drop in immediate blood pressure. At 10 s post-stand, the systolic blood pressure difference between BDZ use groups became maximum (21 mmHg); at this point, systolic blood pressure still seemed to be decreasing in BDZ-users, whereas in controls it seemed to be recovering [13].

The association between BDZ and an immediate drop in blood pressure stems from increased venous accumulation due to muscle relaxation. Another possible hypothesis includes possible sympathetic hyporeactivity resulting from regular use of BZD.

Long-term use of BZD and Z-drugs was associated with lower DBP and SBP in older people, but not in younger people [14].

5.4 Deprescription of Benzodiazepines and Z-Drugs

When BZD and/or Z-drugs are not indicated (for longer than prescribed, no more than 4 weeks), they should be discontinued.

To avoid withdrawal with worsening symptoms of insomnia or anxiety, or other common withdrawal symptoms like irritability, restlessness, sweating, headache, muscle cramps, gastrointestinal discomfort, gradual reduction is required [15, 16].

Tapering will reduce but may not eliminate withdrawal symptoms. Deprescribing is defined as "the withdrawal of an inappropriate medicinal product, supervised by a healthcare professional to manage polypharmacy and improve outcomes" [17].

The goal of deprescribing is to reduce the burden and harm of medication while maintaining or improving patients' quality of life.

Expert consensus criteria strongly discourage the use of BZD in older people, especially when used for more than 4 weeks [18]."

BZD should be discontinued in a staggered manner, gradually reducing the dose. "For example, 25% reduction every 2 weeks and a slower taper of 12.5% every 2 weeks near the end of stopping, were used successfully in clinical trials." Switching to long-acting BZD (e.g., diazepam) has not been shown to reduce incidence of withdrawal symptoms or improve cessation rates more than tapering shorter-acting BZD does. Patients using lower doses at baseline and using BZD for a shorter duration tend to have greater cessation rates and lower risk of restarting use of their BZD. When deciding on tapering doses and rates, consider using a slower rate with those more likely to have a higher risk of relapse (e.g., long-term use or history of psychological distress). When withdrawal symptoms occur, they are mild and short term (lasting a few days and up to approximately 4 weeks). In studies detailing benzodiazepine withdrawal symptoms, such symptoms tend to appear and peak more quickly (1–2 days) and be more severe with abruptly stopping short-acting benzodiazepines compared with after tapering long-acting benzodiazepines (4–10 days). "While common, resulting insomnia is typically mild, and patients should be assured that there is no difference in insomnia compared with usual care or continuation of BZD at 12 months." (K Pottie et al. 2018) Deprescribing benzodiazepine receptor agonists).

5.5 Therapeutic Concepts with Psychoactive Drugs

5.5.1 Possible Mechanisms by Which Psychotropic Drugs Can Cause Falls

Psychotropic drugs are specific drugs that act on various types of receptors, transporters, or enzymes in the CNS [19].

By interacting with them, most antagonize the effect of excitatory neurotransmitters or mimic inhibitory ones by causing depression of CNS activity. Simplifying, the therapeutic effectiveness lies in improving a type of neurotransmission supposedly responsible for the disease, correcting abnormal electrical activity, and/or returning neurotrophic activity in certain areas of the brain, secondarily affecting other neurotransmissions generating many adverse effects both central and peripheral. Like this:

- Typical (haloperidol) and atypical (quetiapine, risperidone) antipsychotics can induce falls by antagonizing central histaminergic H1 receptors which causes sedation, hyporeflexia, and muscle hypotonia, by blocking dopaminergic D2 receptors in the nigrostriatal pathway which causes gait disorders to a greater or lesser degree, and some, by blocking adrenergic alpha1 receptors of the vasculature. These are all causes of orthostatic hypotension. (Fraser LA, Liu K, Naylor KL, et al. Falls and fractures with atypical antipsychotic medication use: A population-based cohort study [19, 20].
- Tricyclic antidepressants (amitriptyline) cause falls since they are chemically related to typical antipsychotics, which block H1 and alpha1 receptor. They are

also arrhythmogenic and can lead to syncopal episodes. Selective serotonin reuptake inhibitors (SSRIs, fluoxetine, escitalopram) may be safer as they have no direct effects on the above receptors; however, as a group effect they produce hypodopaminergia which could affect gait.
- Anticonvulsants (carbamazepine, phenobarbital, lamotrigine, pregabalin) and mood stabilizers (valproate) by various mechanisms (GABAergic potentiation, glutamatergic inhibition, decreased excitability and nerve conduction) can also precipitate falls by affecting balance and posture.
- Finally, melatonin and carbamazepine (the former by an unclear mechanism and the latter by inducing vitamin D catabolism) may have deleterious effects on bone mass and predispose to falls due to hip fracture by aggravating the osteopenia characteristic of old age.

5.6 Other No Less Important Contributions

Older adults are a special population vulnerable due to the physiological changes that occur over the years. Such changes are presented as non-modifiable (and possibly cumulative) risk factors for the various disorders that may occur at later ages. Therefore, the use of drugs in old age is always associated with potential adverse effects different from those that would be seen at other times of life, and among which are situations that lead to falls, due to changes in the pharmacodynamics and pharmacokinetics that age and multimorbidity impose. At the same time, dangerous interactions are more common due to the characteristic polypharmacy. For example:

- Pharmacodynamics in the aging brain leads to increased sensitivity to centrally acting agents which can generate confusional syndromes or, in the case of benzodiazepines, paradoxical responses. The reduction of total body water favors the accumulation of fat-soluble drugs, enhancing their effects, or favoring certain types of toxicity. In turn, autonomic dysregulation in advanced ages may predispose to syncopal episodes due to cerebral hypoflow that may be aggravated by alpha1 blockers and other sympatholytics. The prevalence of orthostatic hypotension is shown to increase from 15% to 26% with advancing age, perhaps associated with fewer beta-family receptors and decreased function, resulting in a weaker response to catecholamines.

In any treatment, two needs must prevail, adherence-effectiveness, and maximum safety. By choosing reliably proven drugs for the pathology to be treated and in a pharmaceutical form appropriate to the person, the first need will be achieved. While through a pharmacological anamnesis that rules out dangerous interactions and the clinical or biochemical investigation of early sign-symptomatology that warns about adverse effects, the second will be achieved.

Geriatric treatments are usually chronic or long term. Therefore, the problems associated with them are common and the risk of falling into underdosage causing ineffectiveness or overdosage causing intoxication is great. Like this:

- Errors in prescribing at the beginning of treatment arise from not considering the pathophysiological changes that old age brings. Drugs are chosen that, due to their physicochemical characteristics or pharmacokinetics, are not well distributed, are poorly metabolized or accumulate more, hindering titration and response.
- Communication errors arise from poor empathy between the medical group-caregivers-relatives-patient or among health personnel, translating into a bad instructive message about what should be done during treatment and how to protect the patient from adverse effects or particular situations such as falls.
- Administration-dosing errors arise from poor information about what dose to take and at what times they are often calculated or written incorrectly, what are the titration periods, and whether the medication can be administered concomitantly or not with others or with food. All this can cause psychic or physical discomfort that leads to loss of adhesion.

To all the above is added the prescriptive cascade: an iatrogenic situation generated due to medical ignorance where an adverse effect is confused by health personnel with a new morbid situation and a new drug is added for treatment. Metoclopramide, antihistamines, anticonvulsants, and anticholinergics are the most common drugs involved in the prescriptive cascades and can pharmacodynamically potentiate the effects of the psychotropic drugs described.

5.7 Conclusions

Throughout this review, we have been indicated the potential of certain psychotropic drugs, such as antipsychotics, antidepressants, hypnosedants, anxiolytics, and anticonvulsants, to cause falls in the elderly population. Such potentiality is manifested by the greater risk of suffering from them among those who consume such molecules compared to those who do not.

It has also been indicated what would be the mechanisms by which these drugs cause falls and that other elements, such as morbid situations, physiopathological changes, drug interactions, and errors during treatments, can potentiate such situations.

Obviously, the main objective is to achieve primary prevention among the elderly population and reduce the probability of falling, especially in those that have to be institutionalized or have been recently institutionalized. When secondary prevention cannot and should not be done, the correct choice of drugs to be used is essential, and always best to be keep in mind that a patient who has suffered a single fall is not the same as one who has suffered many, so a systematic study of the causes, taking into account pharmacological and other causes is warranted.

It may be common that in the face of a fall, anxiety, fear, or depression in the immediate future (surgery, use of wheelchair, or the possibility of institutionalization), a patient must be medicated. Given this, the possibility of a dynamic psychotherapy should be considered to reduce exposure to a psychotropic but keeping in mind its potential on falls. If an antidepressant must be used, it is preferable to use venlafaxine controlling blood pressure or bupropion since they are not sedative.

Before an institutionalized patient, the adequate conditioning of his room is essential when a treatment with psychotropic medication is mandatory. For this purpose, it is imperative to consider that the main character is the patient and not the comfort of the caregivers. Therefore, it should be reviewed if quetiapine prescriptions are really necessary for inducing sleep (to deprescribe it), while considering alternatives such as melatonin and doxepin.

A patient on antipsychotics may develop long-term potentially irreversible tardive dyskinesias. Therefore, the use of aripiprazole should be considered because unlike other dopamine antagonist antipsychotics, this is a D2 partial agonist that exhibits fewer extrapyramidalisms.

Finally, the scenario imposed by the popular consumption of BZD, which generate dependence and withdrawal syndromes is quite eloquent and is the result of the wide prescription they have enjoyed for 60 years due to their greater safety profile compared to barbiturates. However, withdrawing a BZD is time-consuming.

In sum, because falls are a common problem among older people and psychotropic medications increase the risk of falls, these drugs should be considered potentially inappropriate medications. The geriatric population is extremely vulnerable, and although no one doubts that current pharmacology has managed to increase the life expectancy of humanity, its use is not without risks.

References

1. World Health Organization. WHO Global report on falls prevention in older Age. Available from: https://www.who.int/publications/i/item/9789241563536. Accessed 13 May 2023.
2. Haagsma JA, Olij BF, Majdan M, et al. Falls in older aged adults in 22 European countries: incidence, mortality, and burden of disease from 1990 to 2017. Inj Prev. 2020;26(Supp 1):i67–74.
3. Bergen G, Stevens M, Burns E. Falls and fall injuries among adults aged ≥65 years—United States, 2014. MMWR Morb Mortal Wkly Rep. 2016;65(37):993–8.
4. National Institute for Health and Care Excellence (NICE). Falls in older people: assessing risk and prevention—Clinical guideline.
5. Seppala LJ, Wermelink A, de Vries M, et al. Fall-risk increasing drugs: a systematic review and meta-analysis: II. Psychotropics. J Am Med Dir Assoc. 2018;19:371.e11–7.
6. Seppala LJ, Petrovic M, Ryg J, et al. STOPPFall (screening tool of older persons prescriptions in older adults with high fall risk) a Delphi study by the EuGMS Task and Finish Group on Fall-Risk-Increasing Drugs. Age Ageing. 2021;50(4):1189–99.
7. Seppala LJ, van der Velde N, Masud T, et al. EuGMS task and finish group on fall-risk-increasing drugs (FRIDs): position on knowledge dissemination, management, and future research. Eur Geriatr Med. 2019;10(2):275–83.
8. Gress T, et al. Benzodiazepine overuse in elders: defining the problem and potential solutions. Cureus. 2020;12(10):e11042. https://doi.org/10.7759/cureus.11042.
9. Dirk O.C. Rijksen et al. Use of benzodiazepines and z-drugs in nursing home residents with dementia: Prevalence and Appropriateness). 2021.
10. Capiau A, et al. Therapeutic dilemmas with benzodiazepines and Z-drugs: insomnia, and anxiety disorders versus increased fall risk: a clinical review. Eur Geriatr Med. 2023; https://doi.org/10.1007/s41999-022-00731-4.

11. Park H, Satoh H, Miki A, et al. Medications associated with falls in older people: a systematic review of publications from a recent 5-year period. Eur J Clin Pharmacol. 2015;71(12):1429–40.
12. Airagnes G, Pelissolo A, Lavallée M, et al. Benzodiazepine misuse in the elderly: risk factors, consequences, and management. Curr Psychiatry Rep. 2016;18(10):89.
13. Rivasi G, Kenny RA, Ungar A, et al. Effects of benzodiazepines on orthostatic blood pressure in older people. Eur J Intern Med. 2020;72:73–8.
14. Brandt J, Leong C. Benzodiazepines and Z-Drugs: an updated review of major adverse outcomes reported on in epidemiologic research. Drugs R D. 2017;17(4):493–507.
15. Vilaça A, Vieira A, Fernandes A, et al. Characterisation of benzodiazepine use in an older population registered in family health units in the region of Minho, Portugal. Geriatrics (Basel). 2019;4(1):27.
16. Pottie K, Thompson W, Davies S, et al. Deprescribing benzodiazepine receptor agonists: evidence-based clinical practice guideline. Can Fam Physician. 2018;64(5):339–51.
17. Reeve E, Gnjidic D, Long J, et al. A systematic review of the emerging definition of "deprescribing" with network analysis: implications for future research and clinical practice. Br J Clin Pharmacol. 2015;80(6):1254–68.
18. O'Mahony D, O'Sullivan D, Byrne S et al. STOPP/START criteria for potentially inappropriate prescribing in older people: version 2. 2015.
19. Sibley DR, Hazelwood LA, Amara SG. Chapter 13 5-hydroxytryptamine (serotonin) and dopamine. In: Brunton LL, Hilal-Dandan R, Knollmann BC, editors. Goodman & Gilman the pharmacological bases of therapeutics. 13th ed. Mexico City: McGraw Hill Education; 2019. p. 225–42.
20. JAMA Intern Med. 2015;175:450–2. https://doi.org/10.1001/jamainternmed.2014.6930.

Loneliness and Psychiatric Disorders in Older Adults

6

Federico Triolo, Linnea Sjöberg, Amaia Calderón-Larrañaga, and Lena Dahlberg

6.1 Loneliness Definitions, Prevalence, and Risk Factors

6.1.1 Definitions and Measurements

Loneliness has commonly been defined as a negative feeling arising from a perceived deficiency in a person's social relations, that is, when there is a discrepancy between the social relations a person has and the relations that s/he wishes to have [1]. The discrepancy between achieved and desired levels of social relations may concern quantitative and/or qualitative aspects of these relations, for example, satisfaction in how many relations a person has and contact frequency, or the trust or intimacy s/he experiences in these relations [2]. Loneliness is, thus, subjective and thereby distinct from the more objective states of living alone or social isolation, where the latter refers to the actual number of relations and frequency in contacts regardless of the individual's preferred level of social relations. Loneliness is also distinct from solitude, which is defined as a positive feeling (Box 6.1).

F. Triolo · L. Sjöberg · A. Calderón-Larrañaga · L. Dahlberg (✉)
Department of Neurobiology, Care Sciences and Society; Aging Research Center, Karoliska Institutet, Stockholm, Sweden
e-mail: federico.triolo@ki.se; linnea.sjoberg@ki.se; amaia.calderon.larranaga@ki.se; lena.dahlberg@ki.se

N. Veronese, A. Marseglia (eds.), *Psychogeriatrics*, Practical Issues in Geriatrics,
https://doi.org/10.1007/978-3-031-58488-6_6

Box 6.1 Definitions of Key Concepts Related to Loneliness

Loneliness
A result of a discrepancy between one's desired and achieved levels of social relations. Three aspects have been described: • **Social loneliness:** a response to not belonging to a group • **Emotional loneliness:** a response to lack of close, intimate attachments • **Existential loneliness:** a fundamental separateness/detachment from other people and the world
Social isolation
A poor number of relations and frequency in contacts
Solitude
A positive feeling of being alone

Further, different types or dimensions of loneliness have been identified. In the early 1970s, Weiss defined two types of loneliness: the social and the emotional [3]. Social loneliness refers to feeling arising due to an absence of an engaging social network, that is, a lack of a broader group of contacts to which one belongs. A recent conceptual review of research on loneliness in adults found that social loneliness concerns "a sense of disconnection from others", that is, feeling isolated or deprived of companionship, or not having a sense of belonging [4]. Emotional loneliness, on the other hand, is characterised by the absence of emotionally close relations [3], that is, a lack of good quality social relations [4]. An additional type of loneliness is the existential. This type of loneliness has less to do with the evaluation of social relations and more to do with fundamental separateness from other people and the world and feeling psychologically and emotionally detached [4–6], that is, with "the nature of existence and, in particular, a lack of meaning in life" [7]. Another feature of this type of loneliness is the awareness of being mortal [5], and it has been argued that existential loneliness is mostly experienced in life-threatening situations or other kinds of crisis [5, 8]. Consequently, research on existential loneliness has primarily been undertaken in the context of chronic illness and end-of-life care [4].

Loneliness and related concepts have been measured in various ways [9]. Often, loneliness is assessed with a single item measuring either intensity or frequency in loneliness. While this is a direct and easy way to assess loneliness, it is dependent on the respondents' understanding of the concept, and respondents may also find it difficult to admit to feelings of loneliness because of the attached social stigma [10, 11]. Instruments have been developed to measure loneliness in more indirect ways by avoiding mentioning the term. Commonly used scales [12, 13] in research on older adults are the UCLA (University of California, Los Angeles) Loneliness Scale [14] and the de Jong-Gierveld Loneliness Scale [15]. Single items and the UCLA scale measure loneliness as a global phenomenon, whereas the de Jong-Gierveld Loneliness Scale includes subscales of the social and emotional dimensions of loneliness. While research on existential loneliness is less common, the Existential Loneliness Questionnaire focuses on this type of loneliness (see [7]).

6.1.2 Prevalence

Individuals can experience varying degrees of loneliness over the life course, both regarding how intense the feeling is, how often it occurs, and whether it is a situational or a more enduring or chronic experience. This makes it difficult to interpret specific prevalence figures. However, a meta-analysis of the prevalence of loneliness in older adults (60+ years) in high-income countries defined persons as lonely if they in any way answered positively (e.g., sometimes, often, always) to questions on loneliness frequency [12]. A pooled prevalence of 28% was estimated, while sub-analyses found that 8% of older adults experienced severe loneliness, that is, reporting the highest possible category of loneliness. Cross-European studies have consistently found loneliness to be more common in Eastern than Northern Europe (e.g., [16–18]), which was confirmed in a meta-analysis [19].

There seems to be a common understanding of increasing levels of loneliness over time, for example, reported in media. However, research findings reveal a stable prevalence of loneliness, as shown, among others, in a repeated cross-sectional study covering 1992 to 2014 in Sweden [20] and a study comparing the prevalence of loneliness in London 1999 with studies conducted in the 1940s to 1960s [21]. Similarly, studies in Finland have reported limited or no significant changes in loneliness in older adults over periods of 10 and 20 year, respectively [22, 23]. Although the prevalence of loneliness seems to be stable, the demographic changes with ageing populations still mean that the number of older adults experiencing loneliness is increasing.

Importantly, several studies have also reported an increase in loneliness during the COVID-19 pandemic [24]. During the COVID-19 pandemic, many countries enforced restrictions on physical social contacts to prevent the virus to spread. Often, these restrictions were greater for older adults, as they had a higher risk of poor outcomes if infected [25].

6.1.3 Risk Factors

Several reviews have examined factors associated with loneliness, where most of the included studies have been of cross-sectional design [26], which means that no conclusions can be drawn on causality. There has been one systematic review of longitudinal risk factors of loneliness in older adults [13]. This review identified 120 unique risk factors and concluded that the evidence base was broad but shallow, as that limited research had been conducted for most of these factors. In the review, potential risk factors were divided into five categories: demographic, socio-economic, social, health-related, and psychological factors. The following factors had been included in several articles with relatively consistent associations with loneliness: not being married/partnered and partner loss; a limited social network; a low level of social activity; poor self-perceived health; and depression and an increase in depression. In addition, female gender and higher age were found to be consistently associated with loneliness, although only in unadjusted analyses, which means that these associations could be explained by, e.g., higher risk of widowhood and poorer physical and mental health in women and the oldest old adults.

In the context of this book chapter, the findings on psychological and cognition-related risk factors may be particularly interesting. While only examined in one of the articles included in the afore-mentioned review, anxiety was found to increase the risk of loneliness. No association was found between cognition and loneliness in three articles, whereas one article found that becoming cognitively impaired or being persistently impaired over the study period increased the risk of loneliness. Taken together, this review suggests that psychological factors can be risk factors for loneliness, with the clearest evidence for depression [13].

6.2 Association Between Loneliness and Psychiatric Disorders

6.2.1 Association Between Loneliness and Depression

According to the International Classification of Diseases and the Diagnostic and Statistical Manual of Mental Disorders [27, 28], depression is a mental condition characterised by feelings of sadness and loss of interest or pleasure in activities that the person used to enjoy. Depression can also include symptoms such as despair, loss of energy, difficulty dealing with normal daily life, and changes in eating or sleeping habits. The presentation of symptoms can vary between younger and older adults, where somatic symptoms such as fatigue and disturbed eating or sleeping habits are more common in older adults [29]. The intensity of depression varies from mild to major, where the latter is regarded as clinical depression [28]. It should be noted that research often relies on self-reported rating scales, and that these may have to do with depressive symptoms rather than clinically diagnosed depression.

Depression is not uncommon in people experiencing loneliness [30], and there are conceptual overlaps. For example, an item on loneliness is included in a well-established instrument for depression assessment [31]. There are, however, fundamental differences between these concepts, as loneliness concerns how a person feels regarding her/his social relations, while depression is a more general feeling. Also, persons experiencing loneliness usually have a desire to integrate in social relations, whereas persons with depression often do not want to impose their unhappiness on other people [3], and research has shown that the concepts are distinct [32].

There is a well-established association between loneliness and depression: meta-analyses found that loneliness had a significant effect on depression across several subgroups of the population, including older adults [33]. A review showed that loneliness increases the risk of both depression at follow-up and an unfavourable course of depression [34].

Despite these findings, Van As and colleagues [34] conclude that the causal link between loneliness and depression needs to be examined further, and reviews have noted a dominance of cross-sectional studies, which limits the potential to examine mechanisms and determine causal links [26, 35, 36]. Reviews of longitudinal studies have not only found loneliness to be a risk factor for depression [34], but also that depression is a risk factor for loneliness [13].

Cross-lagged analyses, which have the potential to disentangle this bidirectional relationship, have shown mixed findings. Studies have found loneliness to be predictive of depression but not vice versa [32], depression to be predictive of loneliness but not vice versa [37], and a reciprocal relationship of loneliness and depression [38, 39]. A reciprocal effect means that loneliness and depression are likely to co-occur, and has implications for health in older adults [39]. In summary, there is a robust association between loneliness and depression, but further research is needed to determine causality and potentially reciprocal effects between loneliness and depression.

6.2.2 Association Between Loneliness and Anxiety

Anxiety is commonly experienced in old age and is characterised by a persistent and burdensome fear and worry of perceived threats [40]. Anxiety syndromes include disorders such as generalised anxiety disorder (GAD), panic disorder, social phobia, specific phobia, and obsessive-compulsive disorder (OCD). GAD is the most common anxiety disorder in older adults, and the symptoms involve persistent and excessive worry about daily activities and events. The overall occurrence of anxiety disorders is estimated to range between 6% and 12% in older adults aged 65 years and above [41]. As with depression, anxiety is usually assessed in research through self-reported rating scales.

Cross-sectional associations between loneliness and anxiety have been found in a review and meta-analysis in which most individuals were aged 50 years or over [42]. In detail, a population-based study of older Americans found that higher scores of loneliness were associated with higher levels of anxiety symptoms [43]. Similar results were found in Italians aged 65+ years [44], as well as in US veterans, where loneliness was linked with greater symptoms of general anxiety [45]. However, these studies did not adjust for any factors that may influence the relationship between loneliness and anxiety. Nevertheless, a study that did control for additional factors, i.e., depression, low general cognition, being female, living alone or in a rural area, still found higher levels of loneliness to be associated with greater symptomatology of anxiety in Chinese older adults [46]. Finally, a systematic review found a relation between various aspects of loneliness and anxiety during the COVID-19 pandemic in adults aged 60 years or over, while controlling for socio-economics and demographics, as well as mental and physical conditions [47].

Longitudinal studies examining the relationship between loneliness and anxiety, which better allow for causal interpretations, have mostly focused on younger individuals [48] or adults with a wide age range [49]. An exception is a study from

Ireland including adults aged 50 years and over, showing that loneliness and objective social isolation were related to an increased risk of a diagnosis of generalised anxiety disorder after 2 years. Another study explored the impact of loneliness on general anxiety in adults aged 55–96 years during the COVID-19 pandemic [50]. Participants completed up to four pre-pandemic examinations between 2015 and 2019, and COVID-19 data was assessed between May and June 2020. Results showed that loneliness was associated with an increased risk of anxiety, independent of physical activity, sex, full-time employment status, and history of psychiatric conditions. They also found an exacerbation of the loneliness-anxiety relationship during the pandemic, as compared to previous years [51].

In conclusion, there is some evidence that loneliness is associated with greater levels of anxiety in older adults in cross-sectional, as well as a few longitudinal, studies. However, more studies are needed to further explore the longitudinal associations, while controlling for potentially influential factors, in older adults.

6.2.3 Association Between Loneliness and Suicide

Suicide in old age is a major public health issue, as its incidence tends to be highest in individuals over 70 years old in most countries [52–54]. Suicidal behaviour refers to suicide ideation (i.e., the act of thinking about or planning one's suicide), suicide attempts, and completed suicides [54]. Studies aimed at understanding the factors implied in suicidality retrospectively analyse the characteristics and circumstances of suicide cases, in an approach known as psychological autopsy. Such evidence has consistently shown the prominent role of social relations, and their lack of, as a predisposing and precipitating factor of suicidal behaviour, which has informed our understanding of suicide [55].

Among the several sociological and psychological theories of suicide [55], the interpersonal theory of suicide developed by Joiner and colleagues posits a prominent role of social connections in the suicidal process [56]. Specifically, it postulates thwarted belongingness and perceived burdensomeness as two proximal factors that can initiate suicidal behaviour. On the one side, thwarted belongingness captures one's need for connectedness and is conceived to be reflected by both lack of reciprocal care with others and loneliness. On the other side, perceived burdensomeness can be triggered by several stressors, including unemployment, family conflict, and illnesses. When co-occurring, these factors can greatly increase the risk of engaging in suicidal thinking and potentially lead to completed cases if the individual gains capability for suicide through reduced fear of death and/or high pain endurance [56].

Epidemiological evidence has suggested that older adults with poor social life are vulnerable to suicidal behaviour [57]. A meta-analysis exploring both structural (e.g., social isolation) and functional (e.g., feelings of loneliness) constructs of social relations has shown that older individuals with poor social ties are more likely to present suicidal ideation [58]. Sub-analyses aimed at disentangling this finding showed that functional measures of social connections were stronger predictors than structural ones. Perceived loneliness was among the strongest factors, as older adults who reported loneliness were twice as likely to present suicidal ideation compared to those who did not [58]. This finding was consistent with a Swedish cohort of 85-year-olds, in which feelings of loneliness were associated with suicidal ideation [59]. Further, as in younger people, perceived loneliness is one of the predictors of completed suicide in old age [60, 61]. Importantly, both loneliness and suicidal behaviour are linked to depression, which has been suggested as a mediator in a recent meta-analysis [62]. However, most studies included in this meta-analysis concerned young and middle-aged adults [62], and therefore more evidence for older populations is needed, as the association between loneliness and suicide has been also observed independently of depression [61].

Overall, findings of the afore-mentioned meta-analysis support the hypothesis that social connections that meaningfully contribute to individuals' needs and reduce loneliness may exert protective effects against suicidal behaviour.

6.2.4 Association Between Loneliness and Cognitive Decline and Dementia

Cognitive disorders are common in old age and affect the way one thinks, behaves, and interacts. Under this umbrella term, several conditions are considered, ranging from mild cognitive impairment to dementia, and all of them pose great burden on individuals and their families. From an etiological perspective, cognitive disorders are characterised by a complex neuropathology resulting from the accumulation of neurodegenerative, vascular, and inflammatory deficits. Importantly, evidence has suggested that neuropathological processes are influenced by several biological and environmental factors, including potentially modifiable social health aspects of isolation and loneliness [63, 64].

Cross-sectional evidence gathered in a systematic review suggests that loneliness in older adults correlates with worse cognitive function, both in terms of global cognitive function and in specific domains, such as processing speed, immediate and delayed recall [65]. Of note, one study found social loneliness to be more strongly associated with global cognitive function than emotional loneliness [66]. Further, longitudinal studies have shown an association between loneliness and accelerated decline in global cognition, as well as immediate and delayed recall [67–69]. While more recent prospective studies have confirmed such findings, it has been shown that decline in cognitive function is also associated with increased loneliness over time. These results point to a bidirectional association, highlighting how loneliness and cognition are closely intertwined in old age [70, 71].

Several studies have tested the hypothesis of loneliness as a risk factor of dementia. Despite several methodological issues that hamper direct comparison among studies, evidence from large prospective cohorts has suggested that individuals experiencing loneliness tend to develop dementia at a higher rate than those without loneliness (excess risk from 15% to 64%) [72]. Loneliness and dementia appear to be associated even after accounting for social isolation, depression, and other relevant behavioural and lifestyle factors [69, 73, 74]. Interestingly, a Swedish study explored different dementia types over a 20-year follow-up, showing that Alzheimer's disease was associated with loneliness, while vascular dementia was not [73]. Further, evidence from a Japanese cohort suggests that emotional loneliness, and not social loneliness, is associated with increased dementia risk [75].

Although such evidence derives from prospective studies, reverse causality (i.e., dementia or its preclinical phases leading to loneliness) cannot be fully discarded as social withdrawal and related loneliness can precede dementia onset for several years. Thus, research with consistent measurements, longer follow-up periods, and covering diverse populations is needed to confirm loneliness as a risk factor for dementia.

Following epidemiological evidence linking loneliness and cognitive function, recent studies have explored potential brain markers of loneliness. A review of 41 studies compiling evidence from structural and functional brain imaging methods has suggested that loneliness is associated with multiple dysfunctions across different brain areas [76]. Recent cross-sectional studies of cognitively healthy older adults have shown an association of loneliness with cortical amyloid accumulation and tau pathology, two preclinical markers of Alzheimer's disease [77, 78]. Further, a longitudinal study has found that loneliness predicts worse development in white matter hyperintensities, lesions that are an expression of vascular burden in the brain [79]. These findings, although incipient and from mostly small studies, shed light on the potential biological correlates of loneliness, substantiate the cognitive consequences of loneliness, and pinpoint potential biomarkers for research and clinical purposes.

6.2.5 Potential Mechanisms Linking Loneliness and Psychiatric Disorders

Different mechanisms underpinning the association between loneliness with poor mental and cognitive health have been suggested. Although some mechanisms seem to play a greater role for certain outcomes than others, most of them are shared among multiple psychiatric and neurological conditions and cover psychosocial, behavioural, and biological mechanisms (Fig. 6.1).

Loneliness is accompanied by maladaptive social cognition as it comes with a feeling of unsafety, impairs executive functioning, and heightens the sensitivity for social threats in the environment and negative social stimuli [80–82]. Negative social expectations are likely to prompt others to confirm to these expectations, which can lead to a self-fulfilling prophecy and further withdrawal by the person experiencing loneliness [81]. Hawkley and Cacioppo argue that "this self-reinforcing loneliness loop is accompanied by feelings of hostility, stress, pessimism, anxiety, and low self-esteem and represents a dispositional tendency that activates neurobiological and behavioural mechanisms that contribute to adverse health outcomes" [81]. This negative mind-set and withdrawal from social relations could make lonely individuals more prone to, for example, depression [83].

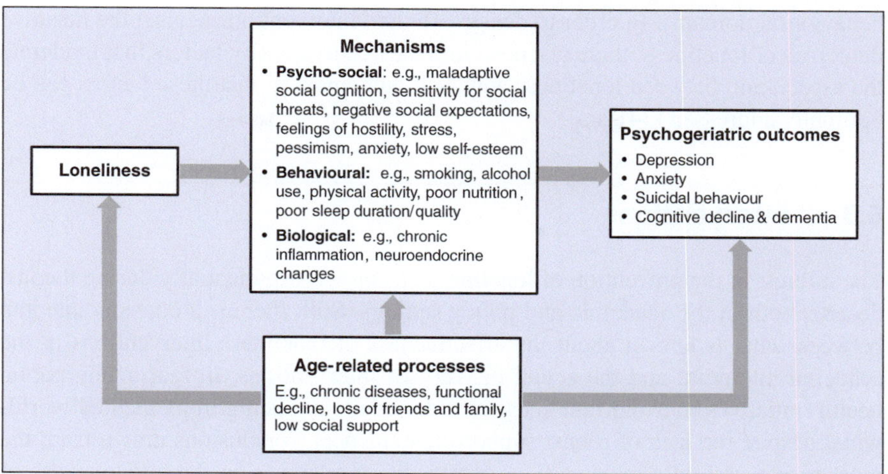

Fig. 6.1 Overview of influences of loneliness on psychogeriatric outcomes through putative mechanisms. Note: Age-related processes may foster both loneliness and mental health disorders, and be mediating factors between these. While this conceptual framework reflects the structure of the chapter, we acknowledge the interrelatedness of phenomena and the possibility of reverse processes, e.g., mental health may be a risk factor for loneliness

Research has shown that loneliness is associated with worse health behaviours, in terms of both poorer health practices such as smoking and alcohol use and lower levels of engagement in health-promoting behaviours such as physical activity and good nutrition [82, 83]. It has been argued that this is due to decreased capacity for self-regulation [81]. It has also been shown that loneliness affects sleep duration and quality, with subsequently poorer daytime function and greater fatigue [81, 82]. Importantly, dysregulated sleep has detrimental consequences for both mental and cognitive health in old age, as it increases the risk for depression, cognitive decline, and dementia [84].

Several biological processes have been implied in the effects of loneliness on mental and cognitive health [82]. Prolonged loneliness has been associated with chronic inflammation due to imbalances between anti-inflammatory and pro-inflammatory factors, which has been consistently linked with both depression and cognitive disorders. Further, loneliness is associated with neuroendocrine changes, leading to dysregulated stress response due to increased activation of the hypothalamic-pituitary-adrenocortical (HPA) and the sympathetic nervous system (SNS), which can in turn foster depression and anxiety in late life [81]. Such neuro-endocrine changes can also lead to dysregulations in blood pressure, which can induce brain neuropathology and, thus, accelerate cognitive ageing.

In addition to the afore-mentioned factors, age-related changes—such as chronic diseases, functional decline, loss of friends and family, social isolation, and low social support—increase the risk of both loneliness and negative health outcomes [13, 39]. This highlights how loneliness is impacted by a multitude of intertwined factors and processes, and can impact multiple biological, cognitive, and behavioural domains. In order to design efficient interventions against the negative outcomes of loneliness, there is a need for research to identify factors that moderate the association between loneliness and such outcomes, so that these factors can be optimally addressed [34].

6.3 Interventions

The interest in the prevention of loneliness has grown exponentially during the last decade, both in the academic and policy settings. Still, there is a considerable gap between what is known about the effectiveness of loneliness interventions in the academic literature and the actual delivery of interventions. In fact, many public health initiatives to avoid loneliness in older adults are being implemented worldwide, despite the lack of robust supporting evidence. Conclusions drawn from the most recent umbrella reviews (i.e., overviews of reviews) on the effectiveness of loneliness interventions have been little insightful and even contradictory [85–88]. However, this does not imply that nothing works when addressing loneliness in later life; it rather highlights the limited scope of existing reviews, which have covered a small range of interventions. Moreover, most interventions have focused on individual services or activities, failing to address the broader challenges arising before older adults are even recruited into the more commonly recognised loneliness interventions [89].

6.3.1 Key Challenges to Addressing Loneliness

Firstly, identifying lonely older individuals is among the biggest threats to the success of preventive strategies. Those who are in greatest need of such strategies are often socially isolated and/or hesitate to admit being lonely due to the stigma linked to loneliness. Ensuring that support services are pro-actively offered to those in greatest need can be facilitated through individual- or household-level data on risk factor distribution, as well as key community members trained to recognise and refer older adults with signs of loneliness to such services [90]. Healthcare professionals such as GPs and social care staff are ideally placed to identify and follow-up lonely older adults and should, thus, be an integral part of interventions. Secondly, understanding the nature of individuals' loneliness is a challenging but essential process, given the individuality and multifaceted character of the problem. While in some cases social isolation is the main trigger for loneliness, in other cases, the pathway to loneliness is unrelated to social isolation, requiring a completely different intervention approach [91]. Guided conversations can be helpful in unravelling the circumstances, needs, and wishes of older persons and can even be supported by the use of checklists [92]. Yet, checklists alone are insufficient to delve deeply into personal issues and potential solutions and should thus be used sensibly. Thirdly, supporting lonely older individuals to access appropriate services is the final key step before embarking on a full-scale intervention. As with many other health problems, there is no one-size-fits-all approach to loneliness interventions, and support services should thus be tailored to meet the specific needs and determinants of individuals' loneliness [93].

6.3.2 Intervention Goals, Approaches, and Enablers

Interventions have mainly aimed at achieving one of the two following goals: (1) to facilitate social bonding (through group-based or one-to-one interventions) or (2) to help people change their perception of loneliness and/or social interaction (Fig. 6.2). Details about the effectiveness linked to specific types of services are provided below.

(a) **Group-based approaches to facilitate social bonding:** Social groups tend to revolve around desirable activities, such as learning or health promotion, instead of directly targeting social contact [94]. This type of interventions is judged as promising by experts [89], and there is widespread agreement on the three main aspects that seem to determine their usefulness [95]: (a) targeted at a specific group and running long-term; (b) focused on a shared interest; and (c) involving older adults in running the activity.

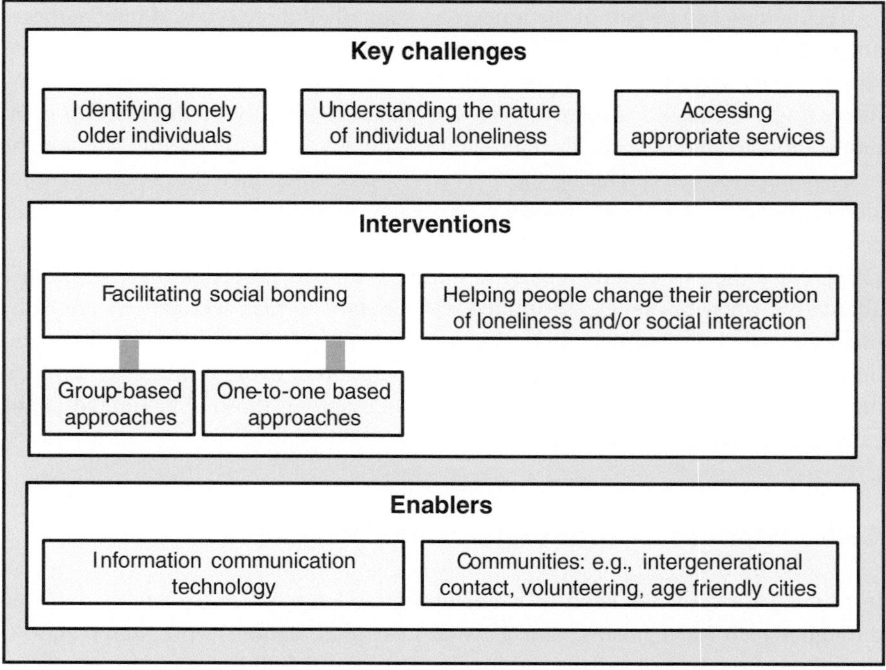

Fig. 6.2 Summary of intervention goals, approaches, and enablers. Note: Adapted from Jopling [89]

(b) **One-to-one approaches to facilitate social bonding:** For those people for whom social engagement in the community comes with practical (e.g., disability) or emotional barriers, long-term one-to-one social support provision at home seems the only solution [89], even if the effectiveness of home visiting and befriending schemes remains unclear [95]. Befriending services aim to match older adults with a worker or volunteer who visits or telephones them on a regular basis. This type of services has evolved in order to increase their efficacy by, for example, involving older adults as befrienders themselves.

(c) **Approaches to help people change their perception of loneliness and/or social interaction:** There is increasing interest in the role that psychological interventions might play in changing older adults' thinking about their social connections, even if the strength of the evidence in this field is still low [87]. The greatest effect on loneliness has been shown for interventions that address the maladaptive social cognition [94]. These psychological approaches are essentially based on social cognitive training and mindfulness. Social cognitive training has shown to avert dysfunctional and irrational beliefs, false attributions, and self-defeating thoughts and interpersonal interactions [96]. Mindfulness is also able to mitigate perceptions of loneliness by bringing one's attention to present experiences [97]. This may, directly, increase older adults' attentiveness to social cues and personal emotional reactions [98] and, indirectly, increase both social cognition [99] and self-efficacy [100].

Technology can be part of the implementation of all three types of interventions, and its role both as a facilitator of social connections per se and in making the provision of wider services and support more cost effective and easy to deliver is being increasingly discussed. Moreover, the use and acceptability of information communication technology (ICT) interventions are gradually increasing among the older population [101]. During the COVID-19 pandemic, there has been an explosion of research devoted to proving whether new technologies, such as video calls, could reduce older adults' levels of loneliness, but the evidence remains uncertain [102]. Nevertheless, experts recognise that ICT support provision may be the best alternative when resources are limited, even if face-to-face interactions are to be prioritised whenever possible [89]. When implementing technology-based interventions, it is essential to consider the target population to avoid reinforcing the feelings of social isolation due to the digital divide among those with limited skills, capacity, or access to technology [103].

6.3.3 Priorities for Future Intervention Research and Action

In looking forward, we need to better understand for whom, in which contexts, through which mechanisms, and at what cost interventions work. Interventions should moreover specifically target loneliness to avoid further confusion by aiming to also address related issues such as social isolation. Subgroups such as first-generation migrants, LGBT+, and older adults with disabilities may require specific interventions to address loneliness and isolation, given the difficulties in accessing mainstream services and their scepticism that these services will meet their needs [89]. Older adults with mental health problems also deserve a specific focus given the higher prevalence of loneliness and social isolation found in these individuals [93]. Older adults living in care homes represent a great challenge too [104]; the most meaningful relationships for them remain those developed before entering the communal living schemes, regardless of the new connections developed [105]. But above all, a whole system response to loneliness is warranted, complementing the focus on the individual with a focus on the community, and emphasising not only on what is delivered but also on how it is delivered [89]. It will be key to support the development of new structures within communities and neighbourhoods for the primary prevention of loneliness in older adults, whether it is by promoting intergenerational contacts, volunteering, or age friendly cities [106].

6.4 Conclusions

Loneliness is associated with an elevated risk of depression, anxiety, suicidal behaviour, and cognitive disorders in older adults. However, for some of these psychogeriatric conditions, such as depression and cognitive disorders, the association seems to be bidirectional, that is, there is evidence that loneliness is both a risk factor for and an outcome of depression and cognitive disorders. For anxiety, the causal direction is more uncertain among older adults, as most research in this population has had a cross-sectional design. For most outcomes, there is a lack of research specifically focusing on older adults, even though the effects and underlying mechanisms of loneliness may vary across age groups. Hence, while there is some evidence for the associations between loneliness and all the psychogeriatric outcomes included in this chapter, further research is needed to examine longitudinal associations, causality, potentially bidirectional effects, and underlying mechanisms in populations of older adults.

Although loneliness is a complex feeling, and different types of loneliness have been identified, these have rarely been examined in relation to psychogeriatric outcomes. Social and emotional loneliness are associated with different risk factors [13, 107], and it can be anticipated that social, emotional, and existential loneliness have different effects on depression, anxiety, suicide, and cognitive disorders. In a conceptual review of loneliness, Mansfield and colleagues noted that most studies focused on social loneliness, and that current measurements either implicitly or explicitly focus on social loneliness [4]. Taken together, this means that there is a lack of knowledge on the potential contribution of social, emotional, and existential loneliness to psychogeriatric outcomes, and that this knowledge gap is particularly large regarding emotional and existential loneliness. In addition, this implies that there is hardly any evidence on the combined effects of different types of loneliness. Research simultaneously embracing different aspects of loneliness is thus needed, as it would increase our understanding of loneliness and its ramifications, and likely translate into interventions of potentially greater efficacy.

The duration of loneliness is likely to influence its impact on health. Chronic loneliness has been linked to slightly higher mortality compared to situational loneliness [108]. However, most of the evidence on the association between loneliness and psychiatric disorders in old age stems from cross-sectional design or studies with short follow-ups, without looking at the persistence of loneliness over time. Indeed, chronic loneliness has shown to negatively affect the body through altered stress and inflammatory response, which can foster the development of mental disorders. More studies exploring the dynamic nature of loneliness in relation to mental health are therefore warranted. Uncovering the long-term impact of chronic loneliness would highlight, even more, the importance of all efforts aimed at reducing it. Similarly, the mechanisms through which loneliness affects health remain to be fully explored. While there is a strong biological and psychosocial rationale that supports the impact of loneliness on mental health in old age, most evidence available so far is purely associational and does not investigate putative mediating and moderating factors. Describing the causal pathways between loneliness and psychiatric disorders will likely provide targets where interventions can be most effective to promote better ageing.

Loneliness is not an unchangeable condition but can be alleviated, also in old age. Interventions that support older adults in being socially connected, either by increasing their actual opportunities for social interactions or by combatting maladaptive social cognition, can reduce feelings of loneliness. But loneliness means something different to everyone given its subjective and multifaceted nature. It is therefore essential that interventions are tailored to specific target groups, considering their specific risk factors and predisposing circumstances, and that they are designed to meet individual needs. Involving older adults themselves in the planning, development, delivery, and evaluation of loneliness interventions can help in the personalisation of strategies. De-stigmatising loneliness will also be key in order to reach those who are in greatest need of help. Along the same lines, endorsing an age-positive approach to population ageing may pave the way towards communities that enable older adults to remain socially connected.

References

1. Perlman D, Peplau LA. Toward a social psychology of loneliness. In: Relationships in disorder. London: Academic Press; 1981. p. 31–56.
2. de Jong-Gierveld J. A review of loneliness: concept and definitions, determinants and consequences. Rev Clin Gerontol. 1998;8:73–80. https://doi.org/10.1017/S0959259898008090.
3. Weiss RS. Loneliness: the experience of emotional and social isolation. Cambridge, MA: The MIT Press; 1973.
4. Mansfield L, Victor C, Meads C, Daykin N, Tomlinson A, Lane J, Gray K, Golding A. A conceptual review of loneliness in adults: qualitative evidence synthesis. Int J Environ Res Public Health. 2021;18:11522. https://doi.org/10.3390/ijerph182111522.
5. Bolmsjö I, Tengland P-A, Rämgård M. Existential loneliness: an attempt at an analysis of the concept and the phenomenon. Nurs Ethics. 2019;26:1310–25. https://doi.org/10.1177/0969733017748480.

6. Perlman D, Peplau LA. Theoretical approaches to loneliness. In: Loneliness: a sourcebook of current theory, research and therapy. New York: Wiley; 1982.
7. van Tilburg TG. Social, emotional, and existential loneliness: a test of the multidimensional concept. The Gerontologist. 2021;61:e335–44. https://doi.org/10.1093/geront/gnaa082.
8. Ettema EJ, Derksen LD, van Leeuwen E. Existential loneliness and end-of-life care: a systematic review. Theor Med Bioeth. 2010;31:141–69. https://doi.org/10.1007/s11017-010-9141-1.
9. Valtorta NK, Kanaan M, Gilbody S, Hanratty B. Loneliness, social isolation and social relationships: what are we measuring? A novel framework for classifying and comparing tools. BMJ Open. 2016;6:e010799. https://doi.org/10.1136/bmjopen-2015-010799.
10. Routasalo P, Pitkala KH. Loneliness among older people. Rev Clin Gerontol. 2003;13:303–11. https://doi.org/10.1017/S095925980400111X.
11. Victor C, Scambler SJ, Bond J. The social world of older people: understanding loneliness and social isolation in later life. Maidenhead: Open University; 2009.
12. Chawla K, Kunonga TP, Stow D, Barker R, Craig D, Hanratty B. Prevalence of loneliness amongst older people in high-income countries: a systematic review and meta-analysis. PLoS One. 2021;16:e0255088. https://doi.org/10.1371/journal.pone.0255088.
13. Dahlberg L, McKee KJ, Frank A, Naseer M. A systematic review of longitudinal risk factors for loneliness in older adults. Aging Ment Health. 2022;26:225–49. https://doi.org/10.1080/13607863.2021.1876638.
14. Russell DW. UCLA loneliness scale (Version 3): reliability, validity, and factor structure. J Pers Assess. 1996;66:20–40. https://doi.org/10.1207/s15327752jpa6601_2.
15. de Jong-Gierveld J, Kamphuls F. The development of a Rasch-type loneliness scale. Appl Psychol Meas. 1985;9:289–99. https://doi.org/10.1177/014662168500900307.
16. Hansen T, Slagsvold B. Late-life loneliness in 11 European countries: results from the generations and gender survey. Soc Indic Res. 2016;129:445–64. https://doi.org/10.1007/s11205-015-1111-6.
17. Myck M, Waldegrave C, Dahlberg L. Two dimensions of social exclusion: economic deprivation and dynamics of loneliness during later life in Europe. In: Walsh K, Scharf T, Van Regenmortel S, Wanka A, editors. Social exclusion in later life: interdisciplinary and policy perspectives. Cham: Springer International Publishing; 2021. p. 311–26. https://doi.org/10.1007/978-3-030-51406-8_24.
18. Nyqvist F, Nygård M, Scharf T. Loneliness amongst older people in Europe: a comparative study of welfare regimes. Eur J Ageing. 2019;16:133–43. https://doi.org/10.1007/s10433-018-0487-y.
19. Surkalim DL, Luo M, Eres R, Gebel K, van Buskirk J, Bauman A, Ding D. The prevalence of loneliness across 113 countries: systematic review and meta-analysis. BMJ. 2022:e067068. https://doi.org/10.1136/bmj-2021-067068.
20. Dahlberg L, Agahi N, Lennartsson C. Lonelier than ever? Loneliness of older people over two decades. Arch Gerontol Geriatr. 2018;75:96–103. https://doi.org/10.1016/j.archger.2017.11.004.
21. Victor CR, Scambler SJ, Shah S, Cook DG, Harris T, Rink E, de Wilde S. Has loneliness amongst older people increased? An investigation into variations between cohorts. Ageing Soc. 2002;22:585–97. https://doi.org/10.1017/S0144686X02008784.
22. Eloranta S, Arve S, Isoaho H, Lehtonen A, Viitanen M. Loneliness of older people aged 70: a comparison of two Finnish cohorts born 20 years apart. Arch Gerontol Geriatr. 2015;61:254–60. https://doi.org/10.1016/j.archger.2015.06.004.
23. Nyqvist F, Cattan M, Conradsson M, Näsman M, Gustafsson Y. Prevalence of loneliness over ten years among the oldest old. Scand J Public Health. 2017;45:411–8. https://doi.org/10.1177/1403494817697511.
24. Buecker S, Horstmann KT. Loneliness and social isolation during the COVID-19 pandemic: a systematic review enriched with empirical evidence from a large-scale diary study. Eur Psychol. 2021;26:272–84. https://doi.org/10.1027/1016-9040/a000453.

25. World Health Organization. Coronavirus disease (COVID-19): risks and safety for older people. 2020. https://www.who.int/news-room/q-a-detail/coronavirus-disease-covid-19-risks-and-safety-for-older-people.
26. Cohen-Mansfield J, Hazan H, Lerman Y, Shalom V. Correlates and predictors of loneliness in older-adults: a review of quantitative results informed by qualitative insights. Int Psychogeriatr. 2016;28:557–76. https://doi.org/10.1017/S1041610215001532.
27. Diagnostic and Statistical Manual of Mental Disorders: DSM-5™, 5th ed. Diagnostic and statistical manual of mental disorders: DSM-5™. 5th ed. Arlington: American Psychiatric Publishing, Inc.; 2013. https://doi.org/10.1176/appi.books.9780890425596.
28. World Health Organization. ICD 11. 2022. https://icd.who.int/en.
29. Fiske A, Jones RS. Depression. In: Johnson ML, editor. The Cambridge handbook of age and ageing, Cambridge handbooks in psychology. Cambridge: Cambridge University Press; 2005. p. 245–51. https://doi.org/10.1017/CBO9780511610714.024.
30. Luanaigh CO, Lawlor BA. Loneliness and the health of older people. Int J Geriatr Psychiatry. 2008;23:1213–21. https://doi.org/10.1002/gps.2054.
31. Radloff LS. The CES-D scale: a self-report depression scale for research in the general population. Appl Psychol Meas. 1977;1:385–401. https://doi.org/10.1177/014662167700100306.
32. Cacioppo JT, Hawkley LC, Thisted RA. Perceived social isolation makes me sad: 5-year cross-lagged analyses of loneliness and depressive symptomatology in the Chicago Health, Aging, and Social Relations Study. Psychol Aging. 2010;25:453–63. https://doi.org/10.1037/a0017216.
33. Erzen E, Çikrikci Ö. The effect of loneliness on depression: a meta-analysis. Int J Soc Psychiatry. 2018;64:427–35. https://doi.org/10.1177/0020764018776349.
34. Van As BAL, Imbimbo E, Franceschi A, Menesini E, Nocentini A. The longitudinal association between loneliness and depressive symptoms in the elderly: a systematic review. Int Psychogeriatr. 2022;34:657–69. https://doi.org/10.1017/S1041610221000399.
35. Courtin E, Knapp M. Social isolation, loneliness and health in old age: a scoping review. Health Soc Care Community. 2017;25:799–812. https://doi.org/10.1111/hsc.12311.
36. Dahlberg L. Lonely and sad and/or sad and lonely? Int Psychogeriatr. 2022;34:613–6. https://doi.org/10.1017/S1041610222000308.
37. McHugh Power J, Hannigan C, Hyland P, Brennan S, Kee F, Lawlor BA. Depressive symptoms predict increased social and emotional loneliness in older adults. Aging Ment Health. 2020;24:110–8. https://doi.org/10.1080/13607863.2018.1517728.
38. Hsueh Y-C, Chen C-Y, Hsiao Y-C, Lin C-C. A longitudinal, cross-lagged panel analysis of loneliness and depression among community-based older adults. J Elder Abuse Negl. 2019;31:281–93. https://doi.org/10.1080/08946566.2019.1660936.
39. van Zutphen EM, Kok AAL, Rijnhart JJM, Rhebergen D, Huisman M, Beekman ATF. An examination of reciprocal effects between cardiovascular morbidity, depressive symptoms and loneliness over time in a longitudinal cohort of Dutch older adults. J Affect Disord. 2021;288:122–8. https://doi.org/10.1016/j.jad.2021.03.081.
40. Penninx BW, Pine DS, Holmes EA, Reif A. Anxiety disorders. Lancet. 2021;397:914–27. https://doi.org/10.1016/S0140-6736(21)00359-7.
41. Skoog I. Psychiatric disorders in the elderly. Can J Psychiatr. 2011;56:387–97. https://doi.org/10.1177/070674371105600702.
42. Park C, Majeed A, Gill H, Tamura J, Ho RC, Mansur RB, Nasri F, Lee Y, Rosenblat JD, Wong E, McIntyre RS. The effect of loneliness on distinct health outcomes: a comprehensive review and meta-analysis. Psychiatry Res. 2020;294:113514. https://doi.org/10.1016/j.psychres.2020.113514.
43. Lee EE, Depp C, Palmer BW, Glorioso D, Daly R, Liu J, Tu XM, Kim H-C, Tarr P, Yamada Y, Jeste DV. High prevalence and adverse health effects of loneliness in community-dwelling adults across the lifespan: role of wisdom as a protective factor. Int Psychogeriatr. 2019;31:1447–62. https://doi.org/10.1017/S1041610218002120.

44. Gerino E, Rollè L, Sechi C, Brustia P. Loneliness, resilience, mental health, and quality of life in old age: a structural equation model. Front Psychol. 2017;8:2003. https://doi.org/10.3389/fpsyg.2017.02003.
45. Kuwert P, Knaevelsrud C, Pietrzak RH. Loneliness among older veterans in the United States: results from the National Health and Resilience in Veterans Study. Am J Geriatr Psychiatry. 2014;22:564–9. https://doi.org/10.1016/j.jagp.2013.02.013.
46. Wang Z, Shu D, Dong B, Luo L, Hao Q. Anxiety disorders and its risk factors among the Sichuan empty-nest older adults: a cross-sectional study. Arch Gerontol Geriatr. 2013;56:298–302. https://doi.org/10.1016/j.archger.2012.08.016.
47. Ciuffreda G, Cabanillas-Barea S, Carrasco-Uribarren A, Albarova-Corral MI, Argüello-Espinosa MI, Marcén-Román Y. Factors associated with depression and anxiety in adults ≥60 years old during the COVID-19 pandemic: a systematic review. Int J Environ Res Public Health. 2021;18:11859. https://doi.org/10.3390/ijerph182211859.
48. Maes M, Nelemans SA, Danneel S, Fernández-Castilla B, Van den Noortgate W, Goossens L, Vanhalst J. Loneliness and social anxiety across childhood and adolescence: multilevel meta-analyses of cross-sectional and longitudinal associations. Dev Psychol. 2019;55:1548–65. https://doi.org/10.1037/dev0000719.
49. Lim MH, Rodebaugh TL, Zyphur MJ, Gleeson JFM. Loneliness over time: the crucial role of social anxiety. J Abnorm Psychol. 2016;125:620–30. https://doi.org/10.1037/abn0000162.
50. Domènech-Abella J, Mundó J, Haro JM, Rubio-Valera M. Anxiety, depression, loneliness and social network in the elderly: longitudinal associations from The Irish Longitudinal Study on Ageing (TILDA). J Affect Disord. 2019;246:82–8. https://doi.org/10.1016/j.jad.2018.12.043.
51. Creese B, Khan Z, Henley W, O'Dwyer S, Corbett A, Vasconcelos Da Silva M, Mills K, Wright N, Testad I, Aarsland D, Ballard C. Loneliness, physical activity, and mental health during COVID-19: a longitudinal analysis of depression and anxiety in adults over the age of 50 between 2015 and 2020. Int Psychogeriatr. 2021;33:505–14. https://doi.org/10.1017/S1041610220004135.
52. American Foundation for Suicide Prevention. Suicide Statistics [WWW Document]. 2022. https://afsp.org/suicide-statistics/. Accessed 10 Oct 2022.
53. Folkhälsomyndigheten. Suicide and suicide prevention in Sweden [WWW Document]. 2022. https://www.folkhalsomyndigheten.se/the-public-health-agency-of-sweden/living-conditions-and-lifestyle/suicide-prevention/#:~:text=Suicide%20rates%20in%20different%20groups&text=The%20highest%20number%20of%20suicides,number%20of%20suicides%20was%20232. Accessed 10 Oct 2022.
54. World Health Organization. Preventing suicide: a global imperative. 2014. https://apps.who.int/iris/handle/10665/131056. World Health Organization.
55. Stanley IH, Hom MA, Rogers ML, Hagan CR, Joiner TE. Understanding suicide among older adults: a review of psychological and sociological theories of suicide. Aging Ment Health. 2016;20:113–22. https://doi.org/10.1080/13607863.2015.1012045.
56. Van Orden KA, Witte TK, Cukrowicz KC, Braithwaite SR, Selby EA, Joiner TE. The interpersonal theory of suicide. Psychol Rev. 2010;117:575–600. https://doi.org/10.1037/a0018697.
57. Calati R, Ferrari C, Brittner M, Oasi O, Olié E, Carvalho AF, Courtet P. Suicidal thoughts and behaviors and social isolation: a narrative review of the literature. J Affect Disord. 2019;245:653–67. https://doi.org/10.1016/j.jad.2018.11.022.
58. Chang Q, Chan CH, Yip PSF. A meta-analytic review on social relationships and suicidal ideation among older adults. Soc Sci Med. 2017;191:65–76. https://doi.org/10.1016/j.socscimed.2017.09.003.
59. Jonson M, Sigström R, Mellqvist Fässberg M, Wetterberg H, Rydén L, Rydberg Sterner T, Hedna K, Lagerlöf Nilsson U, Skoog I, Waern M. Passive and active suicidal ideation in Swedish 85-year-olds: Time trends 1986–2015. J Affect Disord. 2021;290:300–7. https://doi.org/10.1016/j.jad.2021.04.060.
60. Rubenowitz E, Waern M, Wilhelmson K, Allebeck P. Life events and psychosocial factors in elderly suicides—a case–control study. Psychol Med. 2001;31:1193–202. https://doi.org/10.1017/S0033291701004457.

61. Waern M, Rubenowitz E, Wilhelmson K. Predictors of suicide in the old elderly. Gerontology. 2003;49:328–34. https://doi.org/10.1159/000071715.
62. McClelland H, Evans JJ, Nowland R, Ferguson E, O'Connor RC. Loneliness as a predictor of suicidal ideation and behaviour: a systematic review and meta-analysis of prospective studies. J Affect Disord. 2020;274:880–96. https://doi.org/10.1016/j.jad.2020.05.004.
63. Fratiglioni L, Marseglia A, Dekhtyar S. Ageing without dementia: can stimulating psychosocial and lifestyle experiences make a difference? Lancet Neurol. 2020;19:533–43. https://doi.org/10.1016/S1474-4422(20)30039-9.
64. Grande G, Qiu C, Fratiglioni L. Prevention of dementia in an ageing world: evidence and biological rationale. Ageing Res Rev. 2020;101045 https://doi.org/10.1016/j.arr.2020.101045.
65. Boss L, Kang D-H, Branson S. Loneliness and cognitive function in the older adult: a systematic review. Int Psychogeriatr. 2015;27:541–53. https://doi.org/10.1017/S1041610214002749.
66. Holmén K, Ericsson K, Winblad B. Social and emotional loneliness among non-demented and demented elderly people. Arch Gerontol Geriatr. 2000;31:177–92. https://doi.org/10.1016/S0167-4943(00)00070-4.
67. Gow AJ, Pattie A, Whiteman MC, Whalley LJ, Deary IJ. Social support and successful aging: investigating the relationships between lifetime cognitive change and life satisfaction. J Individ Differ. 2007;28:103–15. https://doi.org/10.1027/1614-0001.28.3.103.
68. Holwerda TJ, Deeg DJH, Beekman ATF, van Tilburg TG, Stek ML, Jonker C, Schoevers RA. Feelings of loneliness, but not social isolation, predict dementia onset: results from the Amsterdam Study of the Elderly (AMSTEL). J Neurol Neurosurg Psychiatry. 2014;85:135–42. https://doi.org/10.1001/archpsyc.64.2.234.
69. Wilson RS, Krueger KR, Arnold SE, Schneider JA, Kelly JF, Barnes LL, Tang Y, Bennett DA. Loneliness and risk of Alzheimer disease. Arch Gen Psychiatry. 2007;64:234. https://doi.org/10.1001/archpsyc.64.2.234.
70. Yin J, Lassale C, Steptoe A, Cadar D. Exploring the bidirectional associations between loneliness and cognitive functioning over 10 years: the English longitudinal study of ageing. Int J Epidemiol. 2019;48:1937–48. https://doi.org/10.1093/ije/dyz085.
71. Zhong B-L, Chen S-L, Tu X, Conwell Y. Loneliness and cognitive function in older adults: findings from the Chinese longitudinal healthy longevity survey. J Gerontol B Psychol Sci Soc Sci. 2017;72:120–8. https://doi.org/10.1093/geronb/gbw037.
72. Victor CR. Is loneliness a cause or consequence of dementia? A public health analysis of the literature. Front Psychol. 2021;11:612771. https://doi.org/10.3389/fpsyg.2020.612771.
73. Sundström A, Adolfsson AN, Nordin M, Adolfsson R. Loneliness increases the risk of all-cause dementia and Alzheimer's disease. J Gerontol B Psychol Sci Soc Sci. 2020;75:919–26. https://doi.org/10.1093/geronb/gbz139.
74. Sutin AR, Stephan Y, Luchetti M, Terracciano A. Loneliness and risk of dementia. J Gerontol Ser B. 2020;75:1414–22. https://doi.org/10.1093/geronb/gby112.
75. Shibata M, Ohara T, Hosoi M, Hata J, Yoshida D, Hirabayashi N, Morisaki Y, Nakazawa T, Mihara A, Nagata T, Oishi E, Anno K, Sudo N, Ninomiya T. Emotional loneliness is associated with a risk of dementia in a general Japanese older population: the Hisayama study. J Gerontol B Psychol Sci Soc Sci. 2021;76:1756–66. https://doi.org/10.1093/geronb/gbaa196.
76. Lam JA, Murray ER, Yu KE, Ramsey M, Nguyen TT, Mishra J, Martis B, Thomas ML, Lee EE. Neurobiology of loneliness: a systematic review. Neuropsychopharmacology. 2021;46:1873–87. https://doi.org/10.1038/s41386-021-01058-7.
77. d'Oleire Uquillas F, Jacobs HIL, Biddle KD, Properzi M, Hanseeuw B, Schultz AP, Rentz DM, Johnson KA, Sperling RA, Donovan NJ. Regional tau pathology and loneliness in cognitively normal older adults. Transl Psychiatry. 2018;8:282. https://doi.org/10.1038/s41398-018-0345-x.
78. Donovan NJ, Okereke OI, Vannini P, Amariglio RE, Rentz DM, Marshall GA, Johnson KA, Sperling RA. Association of higher cortical amyloid burden with loneliness in cognitively normal older adults. JAMA Psychiatry. 2016;73(12):1230–7.
79. Duan D, Dong Y, Zhang H, Zhao Y, Diao Y, Cui Y, Wang J, Chai Q, Liu Z. Empty-nest-related psychological distress is associated with progression of brain white matter lesions

and cognitive impairment in the elderly. Sci Rep. 2017;7:43816. https://doi.org/10.1038/srep43816.
80. Cacioppo JT, Hawkley LC. Perceived social isolation and cognition. Trends Cogn Sci. 2009;13:447–54. https://doi.org/10.1016/j.tics.2009.06.005.
81. Hawkley LC, Cacioppo JT. Loneliness matters: a theoretical and empirical review of consequences and mechanisms. Ann Behav Med. 2010;40:218–27. https://doi.org/10.1007/s12160-010-9210-8.
82. Ong AD, Uchino BN, Wethington E. Loneliness and health in older adults: a mini-review and synthesis. Gerontology. 2016;62:443–9. https://doi.org/10.1159/000441651.
83. Quadt L, Esposito G, Critchley HD, Garfinkel SN. Brain-body interactions underlying the association of loneliness with mental and physical health. Neurosci Biobehav Rev. 2020;116:283–300. https://doi.org/10.1016/j.neubiorev.2020.06.015.
84. Wennberg AMV, Wu MN, Rosenberg PB, Spira AP. Sleep disturbance, cognitive decline, and dementia: a review. Semin Neurol. 2017;37:395–406. https://doi.org/10.1055/s-0037-1604351.
85. Fakoya OA, McCorry NK, Donnelly M. Loneliness and social isolation interventions for older adults: a scoping review of reviews. BMC Public Health. 2020;20:129. https://doi.org/10.1186/s12889-020-8251-6.
86. Jarvis M-A, Padmanabhanunni A, Balakrishna Y, Chipps J. The effectiveness of interventions addressing loneliness in older persons: an umbrella review. Int J Afr Nurs Sci. 2020;12:100177. https://doi.org/10.1016/j.ijans.2019.100177.
87. Veronese N, Galvano D, D'Antiga F, Vecchiato C, Furegon E, Allocco R, Smith L, Gelmini G, Gareri P, Solmi M, Yang L, Trabucchi M, De Leo D, Demurtas J. Interventions for reducing loneliness: an umbrella review of intervention studies. Health Soc Care Community. 2021;29:e89–96. https://doi.org/10.1111/hsc.13248.
88. Victor C, Mansfield L, Kay T, Daykin N, Lane J, Grigsby Duffy L, Tomlinson A, Meads C. An overview of reviews: the effectiveness of interventions to address loneliness at all stages of the life-course; 2018.
89. Jopling K. Promising approaches to reducing loneliness and isolation in later life. London: Age UK & Campaign to End Loneliness; 2015. https://www.campaigntoendloneliness.org/wp-content/uploads/Promising-approaches-to-reducing-loneliness-and-isolation-in-later-life.pdf.
90. Florio ER, Raschko R. The gatekeeper model: implications for social policy. J Aging Soc Policy. 1998;10:37–55. https://doi.org/10.1300/j031v10n01_03.
91. Dickens AP, Richards SH, Greaves CJ, Campbell JL. Interventions targeting social isolation in older people: a systematic review. BMC Public Health. 2011;11:647. https://doi.org/10.1186/1471-2458-11-647.
92. Goodman A, Adams A, Swift H. Hidden citizens: how can we identify the most lonely older adults?; 2015.
93. Mann F, Bone JK, Lloyd-Evans B, Frerichs J, Pinfold V, Ma R, Wang J, Johnson S. A life less lonely: the state of the art in interventions to reduce loneliness in people with mental health problems. Soc Psychiatry Psychiatr Epidemiol. 2017;52:627–38. https://doi.org/10.1007/s00127-017-1392-y.
94. Masi CM, Chen H-Y, Hawkley LC, Cacioppo JT. A meta-analysis of interventions to reduce loneliness. Pers Soc Psychol Rev. 2011;15:219–66. https://doi.org/10.1177/1088868310377394.
95. Cattan M, White M, Bond J, Learmouth A. Preventing social isolation and loneliness among older people: a systematic review of health promotion interventions. Ageing Soc. 2005;25:41–67. https://doi.org/10.1017/S0144686X04002594.
96. Cacioppo S, Grippo AJ, London S, Goossens L, Cacioppo JT. Loneliness: clinical import and interventions. Perspect Psychol Sci. 2015;10:238–49. https://doi.org/10.1177/1745691615570616.
97. Creswell JD. Mindfulness interventions. Annu Rev Psychol. 2017;68:491–516. https://doi.org/10.1146/annurev-psych-042716-051139.

98. Lindsay EK, Young S, Brown KW, Smyth JM, Creswell JD. Mindfulness training reduces loneliness and increases social contact in a randomized controlled trial. Proc Natl Acad Sci. 2019;116:3488–93. https://doi.org/10.1073/pnas.1813588116.
99. Campos D, Modrego-Alarcón M, López-Del-Hoyo Y, González-Panzano M, Van Gordon W, Shonin E, Navarro-Gil M, García-Campayo J. Exploring the role of meditation and dispositional mindfulness on social cognition domains: a controlled study. Front Psychol. 2019;10:809. https://doi.org/10.3389/fpsyg.2019.00809.
100. Pandya SP. Meditation program enhances self-efficacy and resilience of home-based caregivers of older adults with Alzheimer's: a five-year follow-up study in two South Asian cities. J Gerontol Soc Work. 2019;62:663–81. https://doi.org/10.1080/01634372.2019.1642278.
101. Choi HK, Lee SH. Trends and effectiveness of ICT interventions for the elderly to reduce loneliness: a systematic review. Healthcare. 2021;9:293. https://doi.org/10.3390/healthcare9030293.
102. Noone C, McSharry J, Smalle M, Burns A, Dwan K, Devane D, Morrissey EC. Video calls for reducing social isolation and loneliness in older people: a rapid review. Cochrane Database Syst Rev. 2020;5:CD013632. https://doi.org/10.1002/14651858.CD013632.
103. Andreasson K. Digital divides. The new challenges and opportunities of e-inclusion. 1st ed. New York: Routledge; 2015.
104. Quan NG, Lohman MC, Resciniti NV, Friedman DB. A systematic review of interventions for loneliness among older adults living in long-term care facilities. Aging Ment Health. 2020;24:1945–55. https://doi.org/10.1080/13607863.2019.1673311.
105. Burholt V, Nash P, Phillips J. The impact of supported living environments on social resources and the experience of loneliness for older widows living in Wales: an exploratory mediation analysis. Fam Sci. 2013;4:121–32. https://doi.org/10.1080/19424620.2013.870811.
106. Lyu Y, Forsyth A. Planning, aging, and loneliness: reviewing evidence about built environment effects. J Plan Lit. 2022;37:28–48. https://doi.org/10.1177/08854122211035131.
107. Dahlberg L, McKee KJ. Correlates of social and emotional loneliness in older people: evidence from an English community study. Aging Ment Health. 2014;18:504–14. https://doi.org/10.1080/13607863.2013.856863.
108. Shiovitz-Ezra S, Ayalon L. Situational versus chronic loneliness as risk factors for all-cause mortality. Int Psychogeriatr. 2010;22:455–62. https://doi.org/10.1017/S1041610209991426.

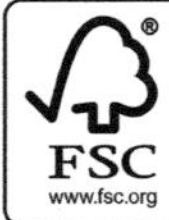

MIX
Papier aus verantwortungsvollen Quellen
Paper from responsible sources
FSC® C105338

If you have any concerns about our products,
you can contact us on
ProductSafety@springernature.com

In case Publisher is established outside the EU,
the EU authorized representative is:
Springer Nature Customer Service Center GmbH
Europaplatz 3, 69115 Heidelberg, Germany

Printed by Libri Plureos GmbH
in Hamburg, Germany